DIGESTIVE DISORDERS

REFLUX

26   Heartburn! (when a hot drink?) clients in also
      water (3/5) Signs. Cut out!
      Treatment

28   Gaviscon (?)

29   CIMETIDINE less powerful than OMEPRAZOLE !!!

INDIGESTION/ULCERATION?

35   Diet high on fat
      Aspirin + every such treatment more slowly Debonair
      Infection
      Stress

☒ IBS ___

      Dealer P 134.

      Diet
      Calcium - Nuts!

Diarrhoea

110   Drug related. Stp a change to avoid reduce
      medicine every time no when   ✳

D0434713

Digestive Disorders

Treatment options and practical advice for sufferers

DR MIKE WHITESIDE

BLOOMSBURY

First published 1995 by
Bloomsbury Publishing Plc
2 Soho Square
London W1V 6HB

A copy of the CIP entry for this book is available from the British Library.

ISBN 0 7475 2090 9

10 9 8 7 6 5 4 3 2 1

Typeset by Hewer Text Composition Services, Edinburgh
Printed and bound in Great Britain by Cox & Wyman Ltd, Reading, Berkshire

Other health books available from Bloomsbury Publishing Plc

Royal Society of Medicine Encyclopedia of Family Health
Dr Robert Youngson
0 7475 2011 9

Bloomsbury Encyclopedia of Aromatherapy
Chrissie Wildwood
0 7475 2085 2

Cancer
What every patient needs to know
Dr Jeffrey Tobias
0 7475 1993 5

Candida
A practical guide for sufferers
0 7475 2025 9

Fear of Food
A self-help programme for permanent recovery from compulsive eating
Genevieve Blais
0 7475 2024 0

Running on Empty
Strategies for coping with ME
Kathryn Berne and Ann Macintyre
0 7475 2138 7

Holistic Woman's Herbal
A complete guide to happiness, health and wellbeing at all ages
Kitty Campion
0 7475 2047 X

Medicines
Third edition
The comprehensive guide
Consultants: Dr Ian Morton and Dr Judith Hall
0 7475 2095 X

With thanks to my
family and friends
for their
love and support.

CONTENTS

1 **Introduction**   1
  ● The incidence of digestive problems ● Why do
  problems occur? ● Healthy eating guidelines

2 **What happens to food when it is eaten?**   6
  ● The digestive process

3 **Alternative therapies**   12
  ● Acupuncture ● Homoeopathy ● Hypnosis ● Herbalism

4 **Heartburn**   20
  ● The reason for heartburn ● Investigations ● Management
  ● Conventional treatment ● Alternative therapies ● Surgery
  ● Conclusion ● Treatment plan

5 **'Is it an ulcer?'**   35
  ● Causes ● Symptoms ● Investigations ● Management
  ● Lifestyle changes ● Conventional treatment ● Alternative
  therapies ● Conclusion ● Treatment plan

6 **'I keep being sick'**   52
  ● Gastro-intestinal causes ● Non-digestive causes ● Periodic
  vomiting ● Investigations ● Conventional treatment
  ● Alternative therapies ● Treatment plan

7 **Reactions to food**   67
  ● Allergy ● Intolerance ● Management ● Summary
  ● Treatment plan

8 **Malabsorption**   73
  ● Inadequate digestion of food ● Disease of the small
  intestine ● Summary ● Treatment plan

9 **Gall stones**   80
  ● Anatomy and function ● Acute symptoms ● Chronic
  symptoms ● Investigations ● Conventional treatment
  ● Alternative therapies ● Treatment plan

10 Constipation 91
● Causes ● Investigations ● Management ● Conventional treatment ● Inappropriate use of laxatives ● Alternative therapies ● Management of specific conditions ● Treatment plan

11 Diarrhoea 107
● Causes ● Diagnosis ● Investigations ● Conventional treatment ● Management ● Alternative therapies ● Treatment plan

12 Irritable bowel syndrome 123
● What is IBS? ● What causes IBS? ● Who suffers with IBS? ● What are the symptoms? ● The four cardinal symptoms ● Diagnosis ● Management ● Conventional treatment ● Self-help ● Stress ● Treatment of the four cardinal symptoms ● Treatment plan

13 Diverticulitis 151
● Symptoms ● Investigations ● Conventional treatment ● Alternative therapies ● Treatment plan

14 Inflammatory bowel disease 161
● Ulcerative colitis ● Crohn's disease ● Treatment plan

15 'Why does my tummy hurt?' 171
● Manifestations of abdominal pain

16 Cancer 176
● Warning signs ● Causes ● Prevention ● Screening ● Treatment ● Positive thinking ● Conclusion

17 'Oh my aching piles!' 185
● What are piles and how are they formed? ● Symptoms ● Investigations ● Conventional treatment ● Alternative therapies ● Treatment plan

18 Common questions about digestive disorders 196

Useful addresses 213

Index 215

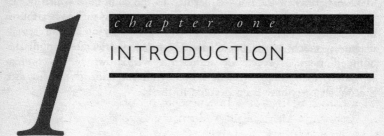

chapter one

INTRODUCTION

'*I'm so sorry but we'll have to cancel our dinner together tonight because my husband is ill in bed with acute attacks of diarrhoea and vomiting.*'

'*I'll not be able to come on the trip today Betty, I've developed this terrible pain in my stomach.*'

'*This wind is awful, doctor. Is there anything I can take for it?*'

These are just three of the commonly occurring situations where something upsets our digestive systems enough to disturb normal day to day living. All of us are affected by digestive disorders at some time in our lives and it always seems to be when we have some important social or business function to attend.

The digestive system, or gastro-intestinal tract, stretches from the mouth to the anus (in other words from where food enters the body, to where it leaves). Disorders of this system include a range of common minor problems such as infections and wind, more significant ailments like stomach ulcers, irritable bowel syndrome and piles, through to major conditions including ulcerative colitis and cancer.

The aim of this book is to provide you with an accurate description of your particular problem, placing the emphasis on simple methods of diagnosis, whether investigations are needed and a comprehensive account of the treatment options available. To help you identify more easily your own problem, each condition is illustrated by typical cases I have seen in my surgery. Over fifteen years of experience as a general practitioner has taught me which treatments are most effective in each situation.

The majority of the book is devoted to the conditions which occur most frequently. As most people experience symptoms such as heartburn or abdominal pain without necessarily being aware of the actual diagnosis, much of the book adopts a problem-orientated approach. Some illnesses, however, are sufficiently well-known to be covered separately, for example irritable bowel syndrome and diverticulitis, so specific chapters have been devoted to these.

The incidence of digestive problems

It is all too easy to think you are the only one afflicted with a digestive disorder, but don't worry! It has been estimated that, at any one time, approximately one in eight people in Britain are suffering from a digestive problem. One in five consultations in my surgery and one in three home visits are for this very reason. The table below shows the main diagnoses in percentage terms:

Acute infections (diarrhoea and vomiting)	33%
Heartburn	15%
Indigestion	12%
Constipation	10%
Abdominal pain	10%
Irritable bowel syndrome	8%
Piles	6%
Others	6%

While specific diagnosis is important, the vital factor is correct treatment and the quickest possible recovery. Most of us are not keen, nowadays, to take large doses of modern drugs, unless they are virtually guaranteed to work. Throughout this book, I have therefore looked at the different treatment options available, both conventional and alternative. In my experience, the most effective approach combines both and this has in fact proved popular with my patients.

Having evaluated the alternatives so you can make your choice, you'll find an easy to follow, step-by-step treatment plan at the end of each chapter. This is important so that when you are acutely ill and don't really feel like reading, you will have immediate help available.

Why do problems occur?

The food you eat supplies the raw materials for building the body and making it work properly. These raw materials are protein, fats and carbohydrates. Preferably, their intake should be balanced, however, it seems the food industry in the West has become highly skilled in convincing us to eat their products, regardless of their nutritional content. This has resulted in a diet which is high in fat and carbohydrates and contains plenty of artificial additives (used to increase a product's colour and flavour).

Our digestive systems were not designed to cope with this kind of sustenance, and inevitably problems result. Too much rich food leads to excess acid production and consequently to heartburn, indigestion and stomach ulcers. This may also put a great strain on the gall bladder and can encourage gall stones to form, with their associated agonising abdominal pain and vomiting.

Food which contains too little fibre leads to constipation, piles and has even been implicated in bowel cancer. Diverticulitis (an inflammation of the lower bowel – see Chapter 13) is common in Western countries but is rarely seen in the developing world, such as rural Africa, where diets are high in fibre. Some doctors also believe that a high fibre diet can protect the body against diabetes and that it lessens the risk of heart disease by lowering the level of cholesterol in the blood.

Not only the type, but also the amount of food we eat provoke digestive problems. Generally, we Westerners tend to eat too much. You might know families in which nearly everyone is enviably slim but, probably, far more where everyone is quite definitely overweight. 'Fatness just runs in our family' they might well say, 'there's nothing we can do about it!' Or they may blame it on their 'big bones' or their 'glands'. And yet being overweight is not an inherited characteristic in the way that blue eyes are, for example, and only very occasionally is it due to any disorder of the glands (an underactive thyroid gland being the one exception). In nearly every case, there is one, simple reason why people are overweight and this is because they eat more food than their body needs.

It all boils down to 'calories in' and 'calories out'. For our bodies to work, they need energy. In a perfect world, we would only eat the exact amount of calories our bodies require each day. If we consume too many, though, we put on weight. If we consume too few, then weight will be lost. It can be difficult for people who are overweight to accept this simple equation and they can be tempted to put the blame on something they cannot control. In the majority of cases, however, corpulent people eat far more than those who are thin. Of course, there are always exceptions – we all have friends who can eat whatever they want *and* stay thin, which can be very irritating!

Undereating, on the other hand, is equally harmful to our digestive systems. The desire to lose some excess weight by adopting sensible eating habits seldom leads to health problems. Crash dieting, however, quite apart from its negative effects on the body in general, can seriously upset the workings of the digestive system, instigating gall bladder colic, generalised abdominal muscle spasm and severe constipation. These conditions occur because a digestive system which is used to a regular amount, is suddenly faced with only very small quantities of food, at far less frequent intervals. In extreme cases, dieting can develop into a condition called anorexia nervosa (a serious eating disorder where the sufferer, usually female, believes she is obese – when, in reality, she is very thin – and avoids food, becoming severely undernourished). Malnutrition and the muscle spasms which occur as a result of this condition, can be severe enough to lead to hospital admission.

Among the latest methods of dieting are low calorie, powdered drinks, which swell up inside you creating a sensation of fullness. Frequently however, they also trap a great deal of wind, inducing bloating, abdominal distension and persistent, embarrassing flatulence. Hardly the most pleasant or effective way to lose weight!

It is important to bear in mind that the digestive system is a creature of habit and likes a constant, regular diet. This is why it can object to a meal out at a restaurant, or play up when on holiday abroad. Changing diet, therefore, needs to be done slowly to allow the digestive system to adapt to different food.

Healthy eating guidelines

When you read, or hear, about diet and health, you will probably have noticed a common pattern emerging. To anyone who wants to work out a new and healthier pattern of eating, these same four rules apply:

- Cut down the amount you eat generally.
- Reduce sugar intake.
- Eat less fat, especially the saturated kind.
- Eat more high-fibre food.

These guidelines will go a long way to help you maintain a healthy digestive system and avoid many of the disorders covered in the following chapters. In treating my patients over the years, I have analysed thousands of different eating habits and have learnt the sort of eating patterns necessary to conquer each digestive disorder. By adopting these habits, recovery is frequently possible, before taking conventional medication.

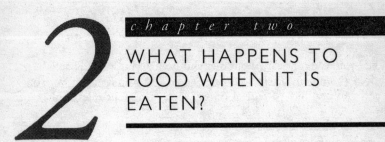

chapter two

WHAT HAPPENS TO FOOD WHEN IT IS EATEN?

M ost of us eat a particular food because of its pleasant taste, but we rarely give more than a passing thought to what happens once it has been swallowed. We take for granted that our bodies will deal with whatever food or drink we put into our stomachs. Yet, each particle of food goes on a fascinating journey through our digestive system. Whether a piece of toast, some fatty bacon, an ice cream, a red hot curry or a gin and tonic, our bodies can cope with it.

The digestive process

Before considering what can go wrong, it is both important and interesting to understand the normal process of digestion.

The initial problem our body is faced with is that the food we place in our mouths is in the form of large chunks. To be of use to us, it has to be small enough to pass through the intestine wall, into the bloodstream. Clearly, one of the main jobs of the digestive process is to break food down into minute particles.

The mouth is the beginning of a very long tube which is called by a variety of names, the most common of which is 'the gut'. Food has to travel about ten metres through the gut before it reappears in quite different form at the other end. The gut lies in the abdominal cavity. This

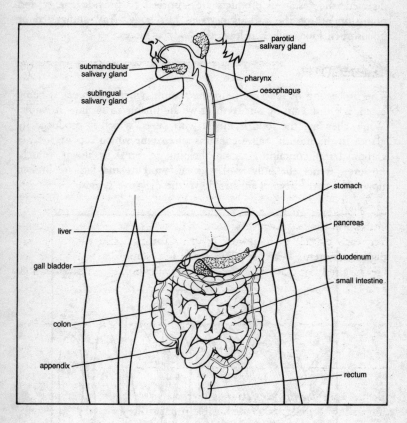

Figure 2.1   The digestive system

is not very large, perhaps about the size of the average shopping bag. To fit inside this cavity, the ten metre long gut is tightly folded.

Between the mouth, and the anus there are several special organs, each responsible for a particular job. Once the food we have eaten has been digested, the resulting products are absorbed to provide energy and nourishment for the various parts of our body. Any undigested or unabsorbed food will then leave the body as faeces.

THE MOUTH

The processing of food starts in the mouth, where whatever is being eaten, is ground up by our teeth, if we are unable to swallow it whole. While chewing, the food is mixed with saliva, which is produced by glands in the mouth. Saliva contains an enzyme which acts on food (a carbohydrate) containing starch, helping to break it down. Starch, however, is not the only food you eat: proteins and fats are broken down by other enzymes further down the digestive system.

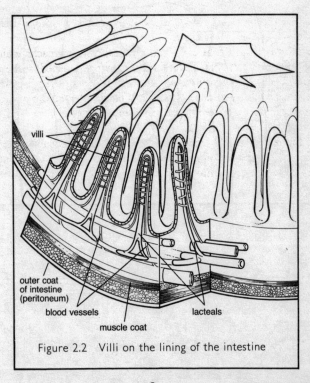

Figure 2.2   Villi on the lining of the intestine

THE GULLET

When food leaves the mouth, it passes down a narrow tube which goes through the chest. This is commonly known as the gullet or the oesophagus. As we are usually standing or sitting upright, much of the passage of food along the gullet is by the effect of gravity. However, throughout the whole length of the gut a set of muscles contract and push the food further on, regardless of our position. This muscular action is known as peristalsis.

THE STOMACH

The gullet passes into the first part of the gut, which is, of course, the stomach. Its lining produces gastric juices which contain hydrochloric acid, the first action of which is to kill most of the micro-organisms present in food. This is vital in raw food (such as fruit and vegetables), as any tiny bugs present would otherwise invade our bloodstreams and cause infection. Gastric juice also contains enzymes to help liquify the food and this process is further enhanced by the stomach wall, which is very muscular and continually churns, mixing the food with the gastric juice. Within two to three hours it is changed into a semi-fluid consistency and is called chyme.

Some animals, such as cows and giraffes, have stomachs which have many different chambers. Here, food is chewed, churned, rechewed and churned again, while enzymes act on it, so it is here that digestion takes place. In contrast, the human stomach is far simpler, acting principally as a temporary store where food is turned into less solid form and where a little digestion takes place.

At the entrance and exit of the stomach are one-way valves. These prevent the regurgitation of food back into the gullet and control the release of its contents into the next part of the gut.

THE SMALL INTESTINE

The small intestine follows on from the stomach. The first part is called the duodenum which gives on to the ileum. In the duodenum, food is mixed with pancreatic juice (a mixture of digestive enzymes secreted by the pancreas); intestinal juice containing several enzymes produced by the gut wall, and bile, an alkaline liquid. Bile is produced by the liver and is stored in the gall bladder. Food which contains fat triggers the contraction of the gall bladder, releasing bile, whose main action is to emulsify fat (i.e. to break large fat droplets down into smaller ones).

At this stage food is ready to be absorbed into the bloodstream and it passes further down the gut into the ileum where this is achieved.

Unlike the stomach and duodenum, it does not have a flat surface, but is lined by many small projections called villi, which greatly increase the surface area of the small intestine.

We all have approximately five million villi, each about 1 mm long. It has been estimated that they provide up to ten square metres of surface area through which food can be absorbed. This is the size of a medium-sized bedroom floor. The area is further increased about fifty times by microvilli which project from each cell on the surface of a villus. Most digested food passes through the walls of the villi into the small blood vessels (capillaries) inside. From here, the blood carries the food molecules away and distributes them around the body.

THE LARGE INTESTINE

As humans have evolved, the digestive process has become more sophisticated and efficient. It will not process anything which it cannot use. Any undigested food will leave the small intestine and pass into the large intestine. It starts with the caecum, attached to which is an irritating little tube called the appendix. In some herbivorous animals, the caecum is a very important part of the gut where a lot of digestive activity takes place. However, in humans, the caecum has very little function and if you have had an appendicitis you will already know how much trouble it can cause.

The main function of the large intestine is to reabsorb the water from the semi-liquid, undigested matter, into the bloodstream. It then passes the caecum into the colon and finally through the rectum to the anus.

When the gut becomes infected, one way in which it responds is to speed up the muscular contractions which move the food along the system (peristalsis). As a result faeces pass through the colon much faster than usual and there is not time for the water to be reabsorbed. The unpleasant result of this is diarrhoea. Constant gurgling in the lower abdomen is indicative of this.

The movement of faeces through the large intestine is made easier if it is full. Roughage, which is provided by a high-fibre diet, is very important in providing the bulk needed for muscles to squeeze against and keep the faeces on the move. Too little roughage in the diet can lead to small hard stools and consequently to constipation.

The digestive process supports huge numbers of micro-organisms or bacteria which are helpful in manufacturing important vitamins.

Although harmless within our guts, if they spread to the rest of the body, they can cause nasty infections. Faeces contain millions of these bacteria and this is why it is important to wash our hands after a bowel movement. Unfortunately gases are a natural by-product of the bacteria's activities and are released from the anus as flatus (wind). A high proportion of flatus is air swallowed while eating, but it is the bacterial contribution which creates the unpleasant smell!

It is essential to realise that our digestive systems work best when we are eating a balanced, well-proportioned diet. All too often, due to our stressful lifestyles, meals are eaten in a rush and often at the wrong time. Furthermore we Westerners tend to overeat and binge, which does not help our guts to function properly. Ideally, we should eat smaller amounts, more often. No single food is, in itself, especially good – or especially bad – for you, no matter what the food advertisers say. A healthy diet does not mean giving up anything you enjoy, or forcing yourself to eat anything you dislike. It is often merely a question of shifting the balance. We must also remember we are not machines – some foods will suit some people but not others.

SUMMARY

As food is taken in, it passes through the digestive system where it is broken down by various processes and absorbed into the bloodstream. Any undigested food passes through the large intestine to the anus, where it is expelled as faeces. The gut is divided into several specialised parts, each with a vital function in the process of digestion. What can go wrong with this process is discussed in the following chapters.

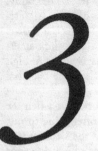

chapter three

ALTERNATIVE
THERAPIES

‹ You're not sticking any needles in me doctor! ›

I will always remember this patient's response to my suggestion of acupuncture. She was the first patient I had suggested this treatment option to and it was only when I explained the theory to her that she was ready to try this method of treatment.

For each condition in this book, I have explained the conventional and alternative treatments available and how they can be used together. These include acupuncture, homoeopathy, hypnosis and herbal medicine. I use all of these treatments at my surgery, but am sensitive to the fact that they are new techniques for many of my patients. To avoid describing the theory every time I recommend them in this book, they are fully described in this chapter and you may find it useful to refer back whenever necessary.

Acupuncture

Most people know that acupuncture is used for pain relief but it is also effective in a wide range of illnesses and in particular those affecting the digestive system. In fact, approximately half the world's population is treated by acupuncture.

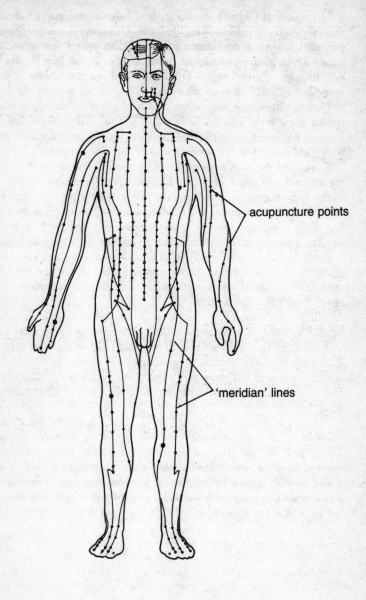

acupuncture points

'meridian' lines

Figure 3.1   The meridians

In traditional Chinese medicine, it is believed an energy called *Chi* flows through our bodies, like a life-force. This flows in a series of vertical pathways known as meridians. Each meridian passes through a major organ, which gives its name: the stomach channel, the liver channel, the gall bladder channel, etc. Tributaries and cross-channels link the meridians to each other so that the *Chi* reaches all areas of the body.

During illness, the movement of *Chi* along these channels is interrupted and it is the acupuncturist's tasks to restore the energy flow. This is done by inserting sterile needles into specific acupuncture points, which are located at the intersections of the relevant meridians.

Sometimes the needles only just penetrate the skin, in other cases they are inserted to a depth of several centimetres. The energy is drawn into the body by the therapist rotating the needle rapidly between their finger and thumb. The treatment is virtually painless – the most that may be felt is a slight pricking sensation. The therapist may also apply heat to the needles, a process called moxibustion, to increase the energy flow further.

Acupuncture sessions usually take about half an hour and are normally given in a course of four to six appointments. Only the very lucky experience a cure in just one treatment, although improvement is often noticed after the first session.

While it is obviously impossible (and inadvisable) to go round sticking needles in yourself at home, a technique known as acupressure can be almost as effective and very helpful for rapid relief of digestive problems. Pressure is applied to certain acupuncture points with a finger or a blunt-ended instrument like the cap of a ball point pen. This is maintained for five to ten minutes, during which time the pain or discomfort may disappear.

As each acupuncture channel has a branch going to the ears, it is possible to carry out treatment simply by placing a needle in the ear. While it is not as effective as using the points along the channels themselves, it is nevertheless useful as an acupuncture stud (a small, coiled needle) can be left in the ear between sessions. When the pain starts, relief can be quickly obtained by gently massaging the stud. The points which are relevant to the digestive system are illustrated below.

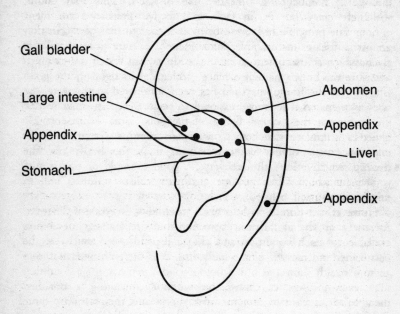

Gall bladder

Large intestine

Appendix

Stomach

Abdomen

Appendix

Liver

Appendix

Figure 3.2   Ear points for digestive disorders

Homoeopathy

Homoeopathy is becoming increasingly popular as it involves taking tablets which have no side-effects. It is a system of medicine where the sufferer is treated by a very small dose of medication that would bring on the symptoms of the disease if taken by a healthy person (literally, the word 'homoeopathy' means 'like disease'). This may sound absolutely crazy but is, in fact, an effective alternative treatment option. The principle of homoeopathy is similar to that of vaccination against a disease, for example polio. Here, a minute dose of polio is given, which is insufficient to cause the illness, but which is enough to stimulate the body's natural defence mechanism to fight off the polio virus. Once the immune system has been stimulated in this way, the body is prepared if it is ever exposed to polio again. In other words: the body, not the vaccine, fights off the polio virus. Homoeopathic remedies stimulate the body's own auto-immune system to fight infection, in a similar manner. Again, it is the body, not the remedy, which effects the recovery. A good example of this is nux vomica, which, if taken in large quantities, causes vomiting but, in minute doses, will help to quell it.

However, the human body is not a machine – everyone is different. A variety of several different homoeopathic preparations are always available for each condition and choice depends very much on the personality and lifestyle of the individual. It is therefore inadvisable to go to a health shop and buy a homoeopathic remedy for a condition such as vomiting or constipation without consulting a qualified therapist. It is easy to buy the wrong one and then assume, quite wrongly, that homoeopathy is not suitable for you. It can be expensive to see a homoeopathic therapist on a regular basis, so I have tried to indicate the homoeopathic preparations for each condition, suitable for a range of personality types.

Homoeopathic remedies can be bought from some chemists and most health food shops. The preparations are available in a variety of forms including tablets, powders, granules, tinctures and ointments. They come in various strengths (I usually prescribe either 6c or 30c). Homoeopathic tablets are very delicate and should not be touched. They must be placed, straight from the bottle, either on or under the tongue, should be allowed to dissolve and should not be swallowed whole. They do not interfere with any drugs your own doctor may prescribe for you and they do not have side-effects. For acute digestive disorders, a week's course is usually sufficient. For chronic conditions however, longer treatment may be necessary.

Hypnosis

Many people find the idea of being hypnotized frightening but this is mainly because of its misrepresentation on television. Hypnosis is one of the most vital and effective ways of treating digestive disorders and one that I use frequently in my own practice.

Most of us believe our conscious mind governs the most important functions, from thought and movement to speech. In contrast, the unconscious mind is commonly regarded as fairly peripheral, fulfilling rather vague functions of which we are not aware. However, the unconscious mind is constantly working and monitoring our physical and psychological functions, from blood pressure and hormone level, to states of hunger and fatigue, even when we are asleep. Never is our unconscious mind more active than with our gastro-intestinal system where it controls all our involuntary digestive processes from the desire to eat, to the urge to open our bowels.

When a patient is under hypnosis, the therapist can communicate with their unconscious mind directly – the very part of the mind that controls the functioning of our stomachs, intestines and bowels.

Many people fear that being in a hypnotic trance will mean that someone else has total control over you. This is a common misconception as you cannot in fact be made to say, or do, anything against your will. The hypnotic state can be described as a halfway state between being awake and asleep. It is more accurate to view it as turning down the conscious, to gain access to the unconscious mind.

Everyone can be put into the hypnotic state if they are willing. The technique is very straightforward: you are asked to focus on a particular object (usually a pen or a spot on the ceiling). This sort of visual fixation tires the eyes and the conscious mind very quickly, allowing the unconscious to take over. Once the patient is in a hypnotic trance the practitioner can suggest changes. Initially, these changes can be those that affect behaviour, such as feeling more relaxed in stressful situations. As the treatment progresses, the suggestions can become more specific, losing the desire to eat excessively for example, eating the right kind of food, or, in anorexia nervosa cases, encouraging the feeling of wanting to eat more.

Treatment usually takes four to five sessions, but some of this time will be spent in learning self-hypnosis. This is particularly useful, for instance, for sufferers of chronic indigestion, where self-hypnosis helps to relieve pain and stave off the desire to overeat.

Finally, it is important to realise that being hypnotized is a very pleasant experience. It will teach you about relaxation and help you cope with living in the modern world. It will almost certainly have a wider application than you ever imagined, when originally seeking treatment.

THE TECHNIQUE OF SELF-HYPNOSIS

As self-hypnosis can be beneficial for several problems within the digestive system, it is useful to learn the technique of inducing a trance yourself. You can refer back to the following description whenever necessary.

The simplest and quickest way to induce a trance is by associating the action of exhalation with feelings of calmness and relaxation. This is first taught by the therapist in the following way:

‹ First, close your eyes. From now on, every time you breathe out, you will feel increasingly calm. As you breathe out, see the word "calm" in your thoughts. Say the word "calm" silently in your mind. As you do this, every trace of tension in your body and mind will disappear. Just let every part of your body relax into the chair . . . calmer and calmer . . . calmer and calmer. ›

This is repeated several times and then, while the patient is under hypnosis, the therapist introduces the idea that, when the patient comes to hypnotize his or herself, all it will take are seven breaths out. With each one, they will become calmer and calmer, until, by the seventh breath, the hypnotic state will be reached. Similarly, waking up can be suggested by doing the reverse (i.e. by inhaling) although, as waking is easier, only three breaths are usually necessary.

Herbal medicine

It may surprise you to learn that the origins of modern medicine, with its heavy reliance on drug prescription, in fact lie in herbalism. Some of the most effective, modern drugs have been refined from plants. Examples include: digitalis (from the foxglove), morphine (from the opium poppy), quinine (from *Cinchona officinalis*) and, perhaps best known of all, aspirin (from the white willow or *Salix alba*).

Herbal treatments have been used for thousands of years and most of their benefits and possible side-effects are well documented. In contrast, many new, synthetic 'wonder drugs' have had limited testing.

The herbalist does not, however, simply hand out herbal medicine rather like a conventional doctor gives out drugs. He or she will also investigate the patient's diet and lifestyle, looking for any imbalance and seeking the underlying cause of the illness. Herbalism considers the patient as a whole person and not simply a parcel of symptoms.

Herbs are very soothing and ideally suited to the treatment of digestive disorders, as they act directly on the gut. They can be taken both for pleasure and for medicinal purposes. The regular use of herb teas and tisanes in replacing coffee, tea and other social drinks, do much to promote good health. Peppermint tea is particularly pleasant and is a great protector of the stomach against excess acid.

Common herbs can be bought from health food shops and are usually prepared as an infusion to be drunk by the cupful. The more modern preparations are in tablet form but in general, traditional herbalists are not keen on these.

Many of my own patients have been cured by herbal remedies, so I have recommended them wherever possible in the following chapters. Indeed, in the rural part of my practice, I meet many old farmers who will not take anything else. One always swears blind that two cups of nettle tea a day has cured his stomach ulcer!

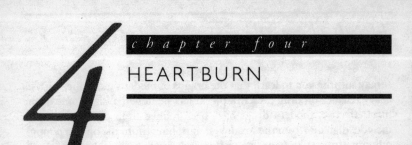

chapter four

HEARTBURN

Heartburn is one of the first problems that can happen as food starts its journey through the digestive system. In its uncomplicated form, heartburn is a burning pain behind the breast bone, experienced soon after eating.

The reason for heartburn

Heartburn occurs quite simply because the acid-tasting gastric juices, which should be contained in the stomach splashes back into the gullet (oesophagus) and irritates its lining. This process is called reflux and, if severe enough, the acid can come back into the mouth, dragging particles of food which has been recently eaten with it. Gastro-oesophageal reflux is nearly always associated with a burning pain in the chest (heartburn).

Reflux is clearly distinguished from vomiting: vomiting is a forceful expulsion associated with abdominal muscle contraction (which is not a feature of reflux). Reflux is an effortless splashing back of the contents of the stomach.

The sensation of heartburn is the end result of reflux, which is caused by several factors. Normally the junction of the oesophagus and stomach has a one-way valve which prevents reflux. In patients with heartburn this valve becomes lax and the contents of the stomach can splash back into the oesophagus. This is why the pain is worse on bending or lying down, because the force of gravity puts further pressure on the weakened valve. A meal which is rich in fat stimulates extra acid production in the

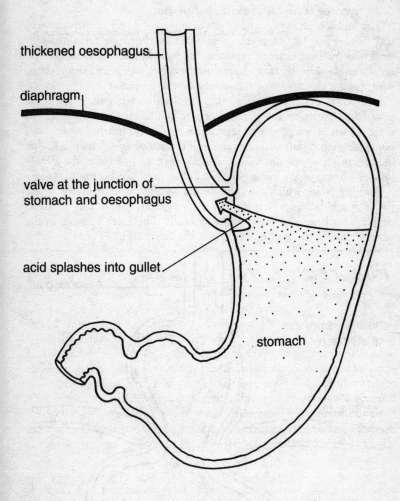

thickened oesophagus

diaphragm

valve at the junction of
stomach and oesophagus

acid splashes into gullet

stomach

Figure 4.1   The mechanism of reflux

tomach and this increases the upward pressure on the valve. The cause of he incompetence of the valve is at present unknown, although it may be lue to hormonal imbalance, as it is commonly seen during pregnancy. Being overweight has also been linked to this.

The lining of the lower end of the oesophagus is very sensitive to acid and bile. There is, however, great variation between individuals in sensitivity to pain, and susceptibility to inflammation and ulceration. Some people may therefore experience far worse symptoms than others, even though the degree of reflux may be the same.

In normal circumstances, food, when swallowed, passes down the oesophagus partly by the effect of gravity but mainly by peristalsis. For some reason, those people susceptible to reflux and heartburn also have poorly developed muscular contraction of the oesophagus. This means that food particles, or hot drinks, can actually stick to, or irritate, the already inflamed lining of the lower gullet, and thus make the heartburn worse.

Another factor which can increase the severity of heartburn is where the stomach becomes very full after a large meal, especially in those people who have a slow-emptying stomach. The extra pressure in the stomach forces the acid upwards into the oesophagus.

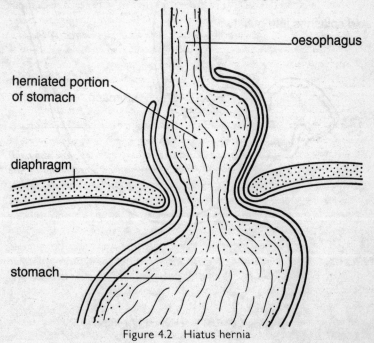

Figure 4.2   Hiatus hernia

Another cause of heartburn is a condition called hiatus hernia where part of the stomach pushes through the diaphragm. (See Figure 4.2). This distorts the valve and allows acid to reflux. Hiatus hernia is actually quite uncommon, although many people will often think they are suffering from this condition when it is simply a case of reflux. Some years ago, an operation was quite common to correct a hiatus hernia, however, nowadays medical treatments are so effective that surgery is usually avoidable. Both heartburn and hiatus hernia are now managed in the same way.

Janet is a fifty three year old woman who came into my surgery with a history of heartburn. Her trouble had started two months previously, at Christmas. While eating some turkey, she had developed quite severe, burning pain in her chest. In fact, the pain was so intense that she had to refuse some Christmas pudding – usually her favourite part of the meal. She was staying with relatives, and they insisted she go and lie down. Unfortunately, this made the pain worse and Janet noticed a taste of acid in her mouth. She even thought she had to swallow a piece of turkey again. Although Janet did not vomit, she felt very nauseous and only obtained relief by propping herself upright with three pillows. Gradually the pain and discomfort subsided and she was able to return to the Christmas festivities, although she ate very little for the rest of the day.

Janet felt well for the next few days but unfortunately the pain in her chest returned at a party on New Year's eve, after she had eaten a large meal and drunk several glasses of wine. This time, she almost collapsed and her friends wanted to take her to hospital. Janet persuaded them not to, simply putting the pain down to the excesses of Christmas. She described the pain on this occasion as starting in the top of her stomach and burning its way up her chest, producing a feeling of constriction in her throat. She was particularly worried to find that the pain also went down her left arm, something she only thought happened during heart attacks. Once again, she felt very nauseous but did not actually vomit. As on the previous occasion, she felt acid in her mouth and some small particles of food which tasted very bitter. At one point, she gave an enormous involuntary belch, and her pain was much relieved by this.

A common New Year's resolution for many of us is to eat less and lose weight. Janet vows to do this each year and, for the next week, did not drink any alcohol and only ate fresh food, which was low in fat. Unfortunately, most resolutions are transient, and by the middle of January she was back on her normal diet and the chest pain returned.

It was at this point that Janet came to see me and I asked her if

23

anything else seemed to bring on the symptoms. Janet is an assistant in a local shoe shop and noticed every time she bent down to fit a shoe on a customer's foot, acid would come back into her mouth. She had developed the trick of bending her knees and keeping her back straight, keeping her head up. This was fine for slip on shoes but tying laces was becoming a nightmare. In fact several customers had asked if she was feeling unwell and her boss was also beginning to notice that something was wrong. Janet was worried that her job would be in jeopardy, if her pain became much worse.

Sleeping had also started to be difficult. When Janet lay down the pain and acid taste returned and she had woken up choking with the sensation of a lump stuck in her throat several times. The only way she was able to relieve this was by sleeping virtually upright, with several pillows propping her up. Her husband was complaining bitterly about this, which increased the tension between them, as Janet had been kept awake by his snoring for years anyway!

On examining Janet, she appeared healthy although quite anxious. A full examination of all her systems was completely normal, including her heart and blood pressure. This was to be expected as heartburn and reflux do not, in themselves, produce any external changes. Although I was almost certain that Janet's pain was due to heartburn, she asked me if she could have some tests to prove it.

Investigations

When the symptoms of heartburn and reflux occur together, then diagnosis is straightforward. Unfortunately, the situation is not always so clear-cut and patients can frequently worry that they may have a more serious condition. Because of its site and the radiation of pain, heartburn can be confused with pain from the heart itself. Heart pain is recognisably more severe and is often described as a gripping or crushing, and not burning, pain. It is frequently brought on by exertion (not by stooping or lying), and is often accompanied by shortness of breath (but no belching or reflux).

Other conditions that can be confused with heartburn include stomach ulcers, gall stones and some rarer, muscular conditions of the oesophagus. So in the small percentage of cases where the diagnosis is not certain, it may be necessary to carry out certain investigations.

BARIUM MEAL

The first investigation involves the use of barium sulphate (an insoluble white compound which shows up clearly on X-rays). It has to be swallowed and is generally considered to taste horrible, but it enables the radiologist to observe the oesophagus and stomach on a monitor as the barium passes through them. Barium studies have two purposes: one is to exclude other disorders of the gastro-intestinal tract (such as stomach ulcers), the second is to demonstrate whether reflux of the stomach contents will occur. The X-ray table is tipped so the person is positioned head-down. If the barium flows back into the gullet, this is proof of reflux. This investigation will also show the presence of a hiatus hernia. However, a hernia itself will not cause symptoms unless it is accompanied by reflux.

Unfortunately, some patients only have intermittent reflux and the radiologist may not be able to confirm its presence, despite using the various manoeuvres which provoke reflux. If this is the case then it is necessary to proceed to further investigations.

ENDOSCOPY

Direct examination of the oesophagus and stomach with an instrument called a flexible fibreoptic endoscope, is a safe and well-tolerated out-patient procedure now available in most district general hospitals. The patient swallows a narrow, hollow tube which has a light on one end and an eyepiece on the other. By looking through this eyepiece the specialist can view the lining of the oesophagus directly and can sometimes even see acid splashing back from the stomach. A snare is also attached to the lower end of the endoscope to allow small pieces of tissue to be taken from the gullet's lining. This is particularly useful to assess how much inflammation the acid is producing.

ACID PERFUSION TEST

This is a relatively new and simple test to prove that the discomfort the patient experiences is from heartburn. A small tube is passed about half-way down the gullet which is perfused (slowly poured) alternately with dilute acid and saline solution. A positive response, indicating oesophagitis (the inflammation of the oesophagus) occurs when the patient's typical heartburn symptoms are instigated by the acid and relieved by the saline solution.

Janet's barium meal showed quite extensive reflux in the head-down position and the endoscopy showed the lining of her oesophagus to be very inflamed. There was no doubt, therefore, that her pain was due to heartburn.

Management of heartburn

However mild or severe the symptoms of heartburn may be, the approach to treatment is the same. Conventional medicine uses three stages of management and the patient's response to treatment is assessed after each stage.

STAGE 1: MODIFICATION OF LIFESTYLE

Simple changes in lifestyle can pay large dividends in the management of heartburn. I go through the following simple, but important, rules with every patient I see for heartburn:

- Weight reduction, combined with the avoidance of tight clothing. This is often all that is necessary to alleviate mild symptoms;
- The avoidance of large meals. Dinner should be eaten several hours before going to bed. Heartburn is likely to happen when a meal is followed by lying down or slumping in a chair, so a good upright posture should be maintained for about an hour after eating;
- The elevation of the bed head on six inch blocks. This can make sleeping more comfortable and is often more effective than extra pillows;
- The elimination of foods causing heartburn, such as cheese, hot drinks, alcohol and fruit juice from the diet;
- Stopping smoking. It impairs the functioning of the valve at the junction of the oesophagus and stomach. It is not sufficient to

simply cut down on the number of cigarettes you smoke – even one cigarette a day can affect the functioning of the valve.

Janet looked after her figure very well and at first glance her weight looked about right. However, on checking the height for weight chart she was about nine pounds above her ideal weight. This may not seem very much. Even so, those extra pounds could have contributed to that defective valve, so I advised her to try and lose a little weight.

A look at Janet's eating habits revealed she liked some cheese and two or three biscuits for supper. Fifty years ago or so, most people ate supper, though nowadays the habit has largely disappeared. If there is one food which is likely to produce heartburn, it is cheese. Janet soon realised that she would have to stop eating it.

As heartburn is such a common problem, I have a local joiner who keeps me stocked with six inch wooden blocks for raising the bedhead. I was therefore able to give Janet a pair with the surgery's compliments. However, any joiner or timber yard will be able to give you these – there may even be some pieces lying around your shed at home.

I knew from my records that Janet was a smoker, so I urged her strongly to give up. This is in fact the single most important contributing factor – all other measures may have no effect, unless cigarettes are binned. You may even risk major surgery.

While women tend to put weight on their thighs and hips, in men excess weight is mainly deposited on the stomach. This greatly increases the upward pressure on the oesophagus, contributing to reflux and heartburn.

Tom a fifty year old farmer fitted this description exactly. When I saw him initially, he was at least four stone overweight and admitted he liked a hearty English breakfast of fresh eggs and bacon, before starting the day. Tom had similar symptoms of pain and reflux and his investigation findings were almost identical to Janet's. To make matters worse, he wore a tight belt, further increasing the pressure on his stomach and oesophagus. However, I suspected their treatment plans would need to be totally different.

At least Tom didn't smoke but he needed to be far more strict with his diet than Janet. A low fat diet was prescribed with, once again, the threat of surgery if he didn't stick to it. Tom also left the surgery with a pair of complimentary wooden blocks for the bedhead.

Tom slept better at night, thanks to the bed blocks. However, his symptoms changed very little over the next two months. He was adamant he had cut down on his food intake but, as his weight had not changed at all, I was a little doubtful about how hard he had tried!

Janet, on the other hand, followed the guidelines very well: she gave up her usual supper, lost five pounds in weight and stopped smoking altogether. Her daily bouts of heartburn had disappeared, which thrilled her. The only problem which remained was that, when she went out to a friend's house or a restaurant for a meal, she would end up eating richer food in greater quantity than usual. The symptoms of heartburn would then flare up and spoil her evening.

SUMMARY OF STAGE 1
1. Lose weight
2. Stop smoking
3. Modify diet
4. Elevate the head of the bed

STAGE 2: CONVENTIONAL TREATMENT

Conventional and alternative medicine have, until now, followed the same path, advocating lifestyle modifications. However, at this stage, they diverge, with conventional medicine turning to drugs. These can be divided into four types:

- **Drugs which neutralise stomach acid** These are called antacids – the white, usually peppermint flavoured, medicines you can buy from the chemist. They have been available for many years and are often all that is needed to treat heartburn and can be taken simply when the pain or reflux occurs. They work simply by neutralising any excess acid that is present and are not absorbed into the rest of the body. Antacids can be supplemented by preparations containing alginic acid (the common brand names are Gaviscon or Gastrocote). These preparations float on top of the stomach contents weighing it down, away from the oesophagus, rather like pouring oil on troubled water.

- **Drugs which decrease the production of acid** These are known as H2-receptor antagonists of which Cimetidine is the most widely used. This group of drugs can be bought without prescription; these drugs reduce the amount of acid produced in the stomach by acting directly on the acid-producing cells. If there is less acid in the stomach, then there is less chance of it refluxing into the oesophagus. This group of drugs are my first choice when prescribing conventional medicines, as they are effective and have very few side-effects.

  More recently, a group of extremely powerful suppressors of gastric acid have been discovered. These have the unlikely name of proton pump blockers. The first of this group of drugs, omeprazole (trade name Losec), is now available on prescription and is used to treat patients whose symptoms are not satisfactorily controlled by H2-receptor antagonists. Omeprazole can also be effective in very severe cases. My only reservation is that treatment often has to be long term and the long-term safety of this group is still unclear as they have only been around for ten years or so.

- **Drugs which reduce reflux** These have been developed to improve the emptying of the stomach, preventing it from becoming too full. They also tighten up the valve at the junction of the oesophagus and stomach. The medication commonly used is called Maxolon but, while it can help to prevent reflux, it does nothing to heal the inflamed oesophagus. Side-effects are quite common and include dizziness and loss of balance.

- **Drugs which protect the lining of the oesophagus** Sometimes the lining of the oesophagus is so inflamed and swollen that simply stopping the acid refluxing is not enough to heal it and heartburn can therefore persist. Carbenoxolone is a tablet which, if chewed between meals and at bedtime, will calm the inflammation. It has to be used with great care in the elderly, as it can cause fluid retention which puts pressure on the heart.

As you can see, a bewildering array of medical treatments are available, both on prescription and over the counter. Initially, my own policy is to suggest alginic acid for a few days. If this is not successful then Cimetidine can be taken twice daily. Something stronger is required only occasionally, in which case I replace the Cimetidine with

Omeprazole. These drugs give effective relief without any significant risks of side-effects in the short term.

> *Tom was very keen to opt for conventional medicine. He had been brought up to believe in them, and didn't want anything to do with herbs or needles, which is fair enough. In his case, heartburn and reflux were a result of a hiatus hernia, so it was likely that he would need the stronger drugs. Even so, I believed it was still worth trying a course of Gaviscon. There was in fact some initial improvement. After two weeks, I added Cimetidine taken twice daily and this eased his pain extremely well. He was still, however, complaining of acid refluxing back into his mouth.*
>
> *I suspected he was not keeping to his diet as he had started to put on weight. I therefore suggested he change his Cimetidine to Omeprazole and the following week he was completely free of pain and reflux, although I am sure he is still eating too much fat!*

SUMMARY OF CONVENTIONAL DRUG TREATMENTS
1. Antacids – taken either intermittently or regularly
2. Alginic acid – either Gaviscon or Gastrocote
3. H2 Antagonists – Cimetidine or Ranitidine
4. Proton Pump Inhibitors – Omeprazole
5. Oesophagus-healers – Carbenoxolone.

STAGE 2: ALTERNATIVE TREATMENT

People are increasingly turning away from modern drugs and their toxic side-effects – who can blame them when there are other, much safer, treatments available?

For heartburn and reflux, I recommend homoeopathic and herbal remedies. I have occasionally utilised both acupuncture and hypnosis, but only where patients have specifically asked me or where the pain has been severe and unremitting.

Homoeopathy
As homoeopathy treats the patient as a whole, the choice of remedy depends not only on their symptoms, but also on their personality and lifestyle. There are four homoeopathic remedies which fit these symptoms:

- **Arsenicum album** is ideally suited to intelligent, sensitive and fastidious personalities, who hate the cold and thrive in warm weather. These people tend to be at their best in the mornings and least active at night. Initially, this remedy can be taken every ten to fifteen minutes for up to seven doses during an acute attack and then reduced to three times daily, with an extra dose at night, if required.

- **Nux vomica** is the treatment of choice for those people who tend to be irritable, like to have their own way, hate to be contradicted and lead a sedentary lifestyle. Their symptoms worsen in the sun and when the weather is dry and windy. On the other hand, they feel much better if it is cool and damp.

- **Lycopodium** (which is derived from moss) is the ideal choice of preparation for those who complain of heartburn and a bloated stomach, which is not relieved by belching. The smallest amounts of food make these people feel full. They tend to be tall, thin, tire easily and may lack physical stamina. Being of an anxious disposition, they feel uncomfortable when surrounded by many people, but dread total solitude. Stuffy, warm atmospheres do not suit them and many find their symptoms improve in the fresh air. Tiring in the afternoon, they are lively in the evenings, and are generally hungry two to three hours before going to bed.

- **Phosphorus** is the preparation of choice for those who have suffered with mild heartburn for several years but whose symptoms have recently worsened. They are bright, imaginative and present a tough façade to the world. They are usually tall and slender and feel better in warm weather and may find relief in having their stomachs massaged.

Janet's heartburn came on about half an hour after eating and left a putrid taste in her mouth due to acid reflux. Each attack was brought on by too rich, or too much, food. She would feel nauseous but not actually be sick and belching relieved the pain.

During her consultations, I noticed Janet looked rather pale and anxious. I know her to be an intelligent woman who shared many of the personality traits best suited to Arsenicum album.

Herbal Medicine

The main herb which helps to relieve heartburn is undoubtedly meadowsweet or, to give it its Latin name, *Filipendula ulmaria*. It has been used for upset stomachs and heartburn since the fifteenth century. Later, aspirin, was extracted from it.

The simplest way to take herbs is by making an infusion, in this case using the meadowsweet leaves, in much the same way as preparing a cup of tea. The fresh herb is preferable, but if not, the dried form is almost as good. Use either 75 gm of fresh, or 35 gm of dried meadowsweet leaves, to which 500 mls of water is added. The water should be hot, but not boiling, as the steam can disperse the valuable, volatile oils. It should be made fresh, each day. The amount (given above) is sufficient to fill one tea cup or a wine glass, three times a day. The infusion can be drunk either hot or cold, though the former appears to be more soothing.

In resistant cases, I have found it occasionally necessary to strengthen the meadowsweet infusion by adding ten drops of liquorice essence per dose. Liquorice, can also be used on its own for heartburn, by sucking the plant's roots, whenever required. It is available from most health shops.

By coincidence, two patients on the same day asked me about the herbal treatment of heartburn. Janet was the first, wanting something to soothe her stomach. The second was a seventy year old woman, Connie, whose memories of her mother giving her peppermint tea when she had been sick as a child, prompted her to seek a herbal remedy for her heartburn. Both Janet and Connie found the meadowsweet infusion very soothing to their stomachs. In fact, Connie was able to use it as her only remedy without disturbing her lifestyle or taking drugs.

STAGE 3: SURGERY

Let me reassure you that surgery for heartburn, as a result of simple acid reflux, is extremely rare. I only mention it here because in severe cases of hiatus hernia, it can sometimes be the only way to relieve pain. The need for surgery, however, is diminishing, as more effective medical treatments become available. If, as you read this, you are one of the unlucky ones waiting for surgery, then please do not worry! It is a most effective operation and only requires about a week's stay in hospital.

It is important to emphasise that the presence of a hiatus hernia is never the sole reason for an operation. Surgery is only recommended in cases of severe pain which cannot be relieved by any of the other treatment methods outlined above.

Conclusion

Our two main cases, Janet and Tom, now only come in to see me every six months for routine checks.

Janet has done very well in making all the necessary lifestyle changes including shedding a few excess pounds, modifying her diet, and has even managed to give up smoking altogether. She is not on any conventional medication and only takes the homoeopathic remedy, Arsenicum album, if she knows she is going out to dinner, or if the heartburn occasionally wakes her in the night. She has taken a liking to meadowsweet and drinks it instead of normal tea. Since starting this treatment regime, she has been virtually free of pain and is very happy in herself.

Tom, although he has done very little of what I have advised him to do, is still well overweight, although he maintains he is on a strict diet! However, he has responded very well to modern drug treatment and his heartburn has virtually disappeared with one omeprazole capsule taken in the evening. If he were to have another barium X-ray it would undoubtedly show his hiatus hernia was still present but this is not necessarily a problem, as long as he is pain free.

As you can see, both conventional and alternative methods can be effective in the treatment of heartburn and reflux.

TREATMENT PLAN FOR HEARTBURN

Symptoms

Refluxing of stomach acid
Burning chest pain

Investigations

Barium meal
Endoscopy
Acid perfusion test

Lifestyle Changes

Lose weight
Stop smoking
Modify diet
Elevate bedhead

Treatment

Conventional medicine

Antacids
Alginic acid
H2-receptor antagonists
Proton pump inhibitors
Oesophagus-healers

Herbalism

Arsenicum album
Lycopodium
Nux vomica
Phosphorus

Homoeopathy

Liquorice
Meadowsweet

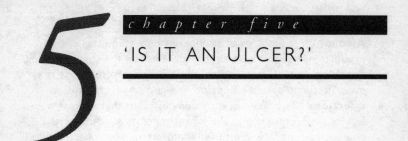

chapter five

'IS IT AN ULCER?'

‹ *Every time I eat I develop this terrible pain in my stomach. Initially it was very mild but in the last couple of weeks the pain has been agonising and has made me sick. In fact it has been so bad that my husband wanted to take me up to the hospital.* ›

Nearly all of us have suffered from indigestion at some time. Indigestion is a term which covers a variety of symptoms which are brought on by eating: heartburn, abdominal pain and wind. Food, as it enters the stomach, stimulates the production of acid which helps break it down. If excess acid is present then the lining of the stomach is irritated, causing pain. If this goes on for a long period of time ulcers (small, distinct craters), can occur either in the stomach or the first part of the duodenum, just beyond the stomach outlet (see Figure 5.1). Indigestion and ulcers can be considered together as their symptoms only differ in severity.

Causes of indigestion and ulceration

- **Diet** Indigestion and stomach ulcers are mainly caused by overeating, or by eating the wrong sorts of food. This leads to excessive production of stomach acid. A diet which is high in fat is most likely to provoke these conditions, although individual foods can also produce this effect, such as spicy food, coffee, cola, cucumber and pickles.

- **Alcohol** Large amounts of alcohol not only stimulates acid production, but also have an irritant effect on the stomach lining.
- **Smoking** As with many other conditions, cigarette smoke is a major factor in precipitating both indigestion and ulceration.
- **Infections** It been recently demonstrated that environmental factors may contribute to the formation of ulcers. Among the possible culprits, are infections. The bacteria, Helicobacter pylori, is now thought to be responsible in some cases.
- **Drugs** Every time you take an aspirin tablet, it will irritate the stomach and may cause a small amount of bleeding. Excessive or prolonged use can eventually lead to indigestion and ulceration. Many of the anti-inflammatory drugs used for treating arthritis can have similar effects.
- **Stress** Stress and tension send the acid levels in the stomach soaring. In fact, indigestion is nervous dyspepsia.
- **Miscellaneous factors** There are a variety of other, minor factors which affect the stomach, including seasonal variation

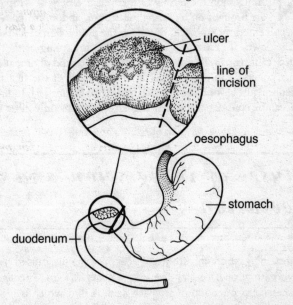

Figure 5.1   Stomach and Duodenum, showing ulcer craters

(ulcers are more common in the spring and autumn). Heredity also plays an important role – you are three times more likely to develop this condition if one of your parents has had an ulcer.

Karen, a thirty four year old woman who is married with two children, also has a job as a saleswoman for a company making hair care products. She is very busy, but by working at a fast pace through the day, she is usually able to be home in time to collect the children from school. This was the first time I had seen her in nearly ten years (other than for her pregnancies) and I therefore suspected that the pain she described just below her rib cage was intense.

Karen always started the day with a decent breakfast, usually cereal and toast on weekdays but she enjoyed a big 'fry-up' at weekends. As she had no fixed lunch break, she rarely stopped for lunch, which frequently consisted of a hastily eaten chocolate bar, sandwich or packet of crisps. Karen's husband is also a salesman but, as he travels all over Europe, he is often away during the week. This meant that Karen took her evening meal with the children, which often consisted of something which was easy to make, such as burger and chips. Her diet, when analysed, was therefore quite high in fat. Looking after two young children with no husband to help during the week, is very difficult for anyone. After her children had gone to bed, Karen liked to sit down with a glass of wine and a cigarette while watching television.

There was no doubt that her lifestyle was very stressful. The company gave her strict sales targets and Karen would constantly worry over these, especially if business was slack. Compressing her day into school hours further increased the pressure, and trying to do her paper work with two young children around, was almost impossible! While Karen's marriage was mainly a happy one, her husband came home on a Friday night, enthusing about his week travelling the cities of Europe, a fair amount of tension occurred between them.

Karen's lifestyle is typical of many of us in these hectic times. With the high cost of living, often a mother has no choice but to go out to work, as well as look after the children.

In Karen, we can see a combination of all the classic contributing factors: high fat diet, stress, cigarette smoke, alcohol and family history (she remembered her father having an operation for the removal of a stomach ulcer). It was therefore hardly surprising that she had developed symptoms of indigestion and ulceration.

SUMMARY OF CAUSES
1. Fatty diet
2. Smoking and Alcohol
3. Drugs, mainly aspirin and anti-inflammatories
4. Stress
5. Miscellaneous factors, including heredity and seasonal variation

Symptoms of indigestion and ulceration

As ulcers are a consequence of persistent indigestion, they are considered together here. The symptoms of each condition differ only in their severity.

- The major symptom is pain in the central, upper abdomen just under the rib cage. The exact site can be identified by the patient pointing with a single finger. The pain often radiates across the chest and back, and is of a gnawing, stabbing quality. Usually the pain comes after eating, when extra acid is produced. Sometimes, however, food can relieve the discomfort as it gives the acid something to work on. In some people, therefore, the pain is worse with an empty stomach, and may even wake the sufferer in the early hours of the morning.
- Vomiting often occurs, which may give rapid relief from pain.
- Heartburn (where acid splashes back into the gullet) is also associated with indigestion.

The symptoms of indigestion and ulceration tend to occur in bouts, lasting from several days to many weeks, interspersed with remissions of many months. However, as an ulcer develops, these periods of remission become shorter. Slight weight loss may also occur.

Karen described her pain as 'like someone sticking a knife in the upper part of my stomach and twisting it'. The pain went straight across her back and occasionally across her shoulder. She felt the pain was related to food and was usually more intense a few minutes after eating. It also woke her in the night and she only found relief by making herself a hot drink and eating a biscuit. At times, she would actually be sick. This had embarrassed her on two occasions, while visiting potential customers.

These symptoms had been troubling her for just over a year, but had become much more severe recently. A full physical examination was normal, apart from some tenderness in the upper abdomen. I was in little doubt from Karen's description of her pain that she had been initially suffering from simple indigestion but that had now progressed to an ulcer.

SUMMARY OF SYMPTOMS
1. Central upper abdominal pain, mainly after eating
2. Vomiting
3. Heartburn

Investigations

Indigestion and ulcers are very common and it is unnecessary to investigate every patient. When the symptoms are typical of these conditions and the patient is under forty it is reasonable to initiate treatment immediately. If the symptoms do not improve, however, investigations to confirm the diagnosis and to assess the severity of the ulcer, are required.

Over the age of forty, investigations are needed to exclude the slight possibility of cancer. Such investigations need not be a cause for concern, not only because it is rare, but also because stomach cancer is not usually painful. It would obviously be wrong to start treatment for an ulcer if there were an underlying malignant growth. The two required investigations are listed below.

BARIUM MEAL

This is the most common investigation in those with a suspected ulcer. It entails swallowing a cup of barium sulphate (a white compound which is opaque to X-rays). A series of X-rays of the stomach are then taken. If there is an ulcer crater present, this will fill with barium and be visible on the X-ray picture.

ENDOSCOPY

Unfortunately about twenty five per cent of ulcers are too small to show up on a barium meal X-ray. This investigation is therefore being superceded by a direct endoscopy (also known as a gastroscopy). While the patient is under sedation, a small flexible tube is passed via the mouth, down the gullet and into the stomach. This has an eyepiece at the top end, and a light and lens at the bottom. By looking the specialist can directly view the stomach lining through the eyepiece. This has the great advantages of revealing: first, whether there is an ulcer present and second how wide and deep it is. If problems are encountered during treatment, a further endoscopy can be carried out to assess progress. The endoscope also has a snare on the end of it which enables a tiny piece of tissue to be taken which is examined under microscope to exclude stomach cancer.

Management of indigestion and ulceration

The aims of management are to relieve symptoms, heal the ulcer and prevent relapse. The approach taken when managing the condition is the same, whether or not an ulcer is shown on the investigations. Even if all the tests are negative, there will still be considerable inflammation of the stomach lining and it is important to clear this up. If indigestion, or an ulcer, are allowed to continue without adequate therapy, then (quite apart from the pain) there is a risk of serious complications. The ulcer may burst, perforating the stomach wall and allow acid to leak out into the rest of the abdominal cavity. This leads to peritonitis (the inflammation of the membrane which lines the abdominal organs) which, if not drained by an operation, can be life threatening. It is also quite common for an untreated ulcer to erode its way through a blood vessel, leading to a haemorrhage in the stomach. As the amount of blood builds up, it causes vomiting (haematemesis). Blood loss may be severe which can be very dangerous.

Managing the disorder is therefore crucial. The first step is to modify your lifestyle.

LIFESTYLE CHANGES

As with any illness, it is essential to eliminate anything in our daily lives that may bring on the symptoms. These include:

- Reducing stress;
- Eating three regular meals a day and reducing their fat content;
- Stopping alcohol intake altogether in the initial phase and, once everything is healed, limiting its intake to no more than two units per day (i.e. two glasses of wine, two single measures of spirits or one pint of beer);
- Avoiding coffee and other drinks which contain caffeine (herbal tea is often quite soothing, particularly peppermint);
- Cutting out cigarettes completely – smoking not only causes stomach ulcers, but also reacts adversely with most treatments, delaying healing. It has also been linked with stomach cancer.

This approach can produce excellent results. Providing the symptoms disappear (for at least a month), nothing else needs to be done. Any recurrences can then be dealt with in the same way. These changes in lifestyle may sound simple but, in practice, can be difficult to achieve.

While it may be difficult to remove the stressful factors in our lives, it is nevertheless still possible to reduce stress levels by learning to cope with them in a positive manner. While a switch of job is not always feasible, it is still worth considering. Often simply thinking about the different options available to you can give you a boost. Try to find something you would really like to do. With a little imagination, it's amazing what can be achieved. For more ideas on how to reduce stress, see the management plan on pages 139–41). You might also find self-hypnosis a useful technique, which is described specifically in this chapter (see pages 45–46) and in Chapter 3 in general terms.

Many people feel they really need their daily dose of caffeine to start the day, but it is important to realise that caffeine is a drug. Alcohol is a relaxant but it can also slow the body's reactions and, in large doses, can even impair health. We all need our treats, but we really spoil our health by smoking. Having seen the suffering it can produce, it is a habit I have come to detest. Even one cigarette a day can cause a stomach ulcer, and prevent its healing.

Most of Karen's stress was caused by trying to hold down a demanding job and bringing up two young children at the same time. Even if she had wanted to, Karen would not have been able to give up her job – as a family, they relied on her income. The stress was compounded by the fact that her husband was away for a good part of the week. Although she was not able to give it up, Karen found ways of improving the quality of her job. She went to see her manager and successfully negotiated a reduction in the area she had to cover. This meant she was not rushing around so much and was nearer to home when the time came to pick up the children. At the same time, she was continuously looking out for an alternative position. She knew she was good at selling, but promoting hair products had not really been her lifelong ambition. Eventually she was able to combine her main hobby, gardening, with her selling skills, working for a company which sold plant feed products to garden centres.

Changing your own habits is relatively simple compared to altering the ways of others. Karen felt her husband Dave needed to do more at weekends to look after the children, as he was away a lot during the week. Dave, however, felt he needed the time to relax. Nevertheless, they eventually reached a compromise: Dave takes the children out on a Saturday afternoon to allow Karen a little time to herself.

Karen also found the other lifestyle changes quite difficult. Three, regular, low-fat meals a day can be nearly impossible to achieve when you are continually on the move. Initially, I describe the perfect lifestyle to my patients and then help them get as close to it as possible. Karen was able to reduce her fat intake simply by cutting out her fry-ups for breakfast and eating wholemeal sandwiches for lunch. Her major problem was the evening meal which she ate with the children who were reluctant to give up their burgers. At least she has reduced the number of chips!

SUMMARY OF LIFESTYLE CHANGES
1. Lower stress
2. Eat regular low-fat meals
3. Initially stop alcohol and then limit it to two units per day
4. Avoid caffeine
5. Stop smoking

Conventional treatment

Until about ten years ago, although it was possible to relieve the symptoms of heartburn, it was very difficult to heal an actual ulcer. At best, the symptoms could be controlled but the ulcer would still eat away at the stomach lining. Eventually the pain would become severe, or a major complication (such as perforation or haemorrhaging) would occur, making an operation unavoidable. The initial surgery was to sever the nerves which stimulate the production of acid. If this was unsuccessful, then the part of the stomach which produces acid was removed (approximately one third of the stomach).

However, good news! Conventional drug therapy is now so effective that I have not suggested surgery as a method of treating a stomach ulcer, for several years. Perforations are virtually non-existent, nowadays.

The course of treatment I recommend consists usually of two drugs in combination:

ANTACIDS

For many years, these drugs have been the mainstay of treatment. While they have no healing effect on the ulcer itself, they can bring rapid, temporary pain relief. They work partly by neutralising excess acid and partly by putting a protective coating on the ulcer. I prescribe them for the first few days until the more powerful medications have had a chance to work. All antacids have much the same effect and can be bought over the counter as well as on prescription.

H2-RECEPTOR ANTAGONIST

The development of this group of drugs, to my mind, stands alongside the greatest discoveries in modern times. Certainly, they have made a major difference in the treatment of indigestion and ulcers and have greatly improved the quality of life of millions of people.

While antacids only neutralise the excess acid in the stomach for a short while, H2-receptor antagonists suppress its production. They work directly on the acid-producing cells in the stomach (H2-receptors), allowing the ulcer to heal.

The most popular H2 antagonist is Cimetidine which is now available over the counter, although it is cheaper on prescription. It is taken in the dose of one tablet (400 mg), twice daily. Approximately eighty per cent of ulcers heal during a six to eight week course of these drugs, compared to only about ten per cent that heal with antacids.

Considering that more than fifteen million people throughout the world have now taken this drug, reports of side-effects have been rare. These include drowsiness, confusion (in the elderly), occasional diarrhoea and skin rashes. However, these are most uncommon and should not put you off trying Cimetidine. Very occasionally, a stronger H2 antagonist is needed, such as Ranitidine, which can be taken in the dose of 150 mg, twice daily. This drug is four times more potent than Cimetidine.

There are other conventional medications available but, in my experience, none as effective as the combination of an antacid with an H2 antagonist. The course of treatment lasts eight weeks, by which time most sufferers will be free of symptoms. As many as one in four patients will have no further problems.

If a relapse occurs very rapidly (which again is uncommon), then it may well be that the ulcer has been caused, at least in part, by bacteria in the stomach called Helicobacter pylori. To treat this, Cimetidine is taken once more, combined with a ten day course of two antibiotics (Amoxil and Metronidazole).

A word of warning: Medication only works if you are prepared to make the necessary lifestyle changes. It is not sufficient to take the tablets, and still carry on eating pie and chips for every meal. You have to help yourself as well.

As Karen was in a great deal of pain, she was keen to start treatment straight away. I therefore prescribed a combination of antacid and Cimetidine. When I saw her two months later, she was a changed woman, free of pain and happy. We stopped the treatment at this point to see whether she was fully healed or would suffer a recurrence.

SUMMARY OF DRUG TREATMENT
1. Initial combination of antacids plus H2 antagonists (Cimetidine) for eight weeks
2. If still pain switch to course of Ranitidine
3. If rapid relapse change to combination of Cimetidine, Amoxil and Ranitidine to eradicate Helicobacter

Alternative therapies

As always, my aim in the treatment of any significant medical condition is to integrate conventional and alternative medicine. Time and again, this approach has produced a more successful outcome than just using either modern drugs or only complimentary therapies.

HYPNOSIS

'No stress, no ulcer' is probably a slight over-simplification, but there is no doubt that stress and tension do play major roles in the production of excess stomach acid. Complaints of butterflies in the stomach, feeling sick with fear or stomachs being turned upside down, are commonly used descriptions of symptoms which may readily presage an attack of indigestion.

It is therefore vital for anyone with indigestion or an ulcer, to learn how to relax. This can be difficult, especially if you have a hectic lifestyle. However, counselling, relaxation tapes or yoga can help. In my experience, hypnosis is the greatest stress-reliever of all. This must be initiated by a trained hypnotherapist but, after two or three sessions, it can be practised at home. Bear in mind that tape-recordings may be advertised as inducing a state of hypnosis, but they are not as successful as self-hypnosis.

Some years ago, I would have described my lifestyle as rather like Karen's – I was always rushing around, desperately trying to fit as much as I could into the day. Since learning self-hypnosis, all that has changed. By disciplining myself to do it each day, I have become much more relaxed.

The main benefits and aims of self-hypnosis are:

- To aid relaxation and reduce the patient's general level of anxiety;
- To reinforce the effect of orthodox, or alternative, medications;
- To help cope with anticipated future events, which may produce symptoms (in this case those of indigestion and ulceration);
- To encourage the independence of the person, so they are in a position to treat themselves.

Most people do not understand how you can put yourself into a trance. The most common worry is that you will be unable to bring yourself out of it. The technique is fully described in Chapter 3. Two sessions are enough to teach someone self-hypnosis and it is a technique which can be used at any time. The people I have taught have become quite adept at using it. One patient of mine used to practise it on the bus going to work every day and, amazingly, always came around just before his bus stop!

Karen was no different to anyone else in feeling apprehensive but, when I had reassured her, she was very keen to give hypnosis a try. She quickly became skilled in the technique. When I hypnotized her initially, I introduced a few suggestions, which she would be able to call to mind when under self-hypnosis.

These were:
- During this sleep you are going to feel physically stronger and fitter in every way;
- Every day your nerves will become stronger and steadier. Your mind calmer, clearer, more composed, more placid, more tranquil;
- You will become much less easily worried, much less easily agitated, much less easily fearful and apprehensive, much less easily upset;
- Every day you will feel more confident, more able to cope with everything that is put before you. All the time you will feel less and less stress;
- At the same time, you will imagine the small ulcer in your stomach, a raw area, roughly the size of a coin. As your stress level gradually lessens, you will visualise the ulcer beginning to heal and feel the pain disappearing. As you become more relaxed you will see the ulcer heal completely.

The technique of visualisation (where you actually imagine you can see healing taking place) has been shown to have positive effects on the immune system. Some people go further and visualise the ulcer as the enemy and their own blood cells as their soldiers, watching them going to war against the aggressor.

Karen was surprised at how easily she became hypnotized, and how simple it was to learn the technique of self-hypnosis. She has even managed to create enough time for it by replacing the half hour she used to have with a drink and a cigarette with a session of hypnosis instead.

HOMOEOPATHY

Ideally, homoeopathic remedies are used in conjunction with H2 antagonists. This creates a powerful combination: medication which acts directly on the acid-producing cells in the stomach, and remedies which stimulate the body's own defence mechanism.

As always, the choice of remedy depends on the condition being treated, but it must also take into account the lifestyle and personality of the patient.

These are:

- Pulsatilla is recommended for shy, gentle people who are prone to tearfulness and changeable moods. Those who are fair haired, prefer cool weather and enjoy the fresh air, also respond well. This should be taken in 6c potency, three times daily, and can be increased to six times per day, if the symptoms are severe.

- Personalities who tend to feel easily depressed, indifferent or worn-out find Sepia a helpful remedy. Such people tend to be averse to sympathy and company, but may dread being alone. They are generally dark haired and have sallow skin. Ulcer symptoms include a continuous empty feeling in the stomach (which may be relieved by eating), a craving for pickles and acid foods, a white-coated tongue, a sour taste in the mouth, flatulence, nausea at the smell of food and less pain when lying on the right side.

- Anxious, thin and apprehensive people who find great difficulty in relaxing should find Argentum nit helpful. Such people tend to be comfort-eaters with a particular liking of sugary food. Symptoms include belching, especially after sweet food, with alternating constipation and diarrhoea. Argentum nit is preferable in the 6c potency (though this is not absolutely critical) and should be dissolved in the mouth, three times a day.

- Graphite (derived from carbon) is ideal for those people who are overweight, whose features are coarse, and whose skin is rough, dry and possibly cracked. They tend to be indecisive, timid, startle easily, suffer from low spirits and may often complain of odd sensations somewhere in the body. It can be taken in either 6 or 30c, for as long as required.

HERBAL MEDICINE

- For simple indigestion, an infusion of centuary, 100 mls or four fluid ounces, taken three times daily, between meals can be effective.
- A few dandelion leaves each day, combined with peppermint tea is also very soothing to the stomach.
- The gel made from the pulp inside of an aloe vera leaf (available from most health food shops) added to milk will aid digestion and calm the stomach.
- Chewing coriander leaves before meals may help to prevent indigestion, chewing them afterwards will ease any discomfort.
- Many cooking herbs are aids to digestion when included in meals: caraway and fennel seeds, marjoram, bay leaves, thyme and rosemary are especially effective.
- For chronic indigestion, it is worth mixing five mls or one teaspoon of powdered slippery elm bark with a little water, to form a paste. To this paste, gradually add 250 mls or eight fluid ounces of boiling water or, if you prefer, half milk and half water. This should be taken three times daily.
- Nervous indigestion can be eased by 45–60 mls (three to four tablespoons) of cold catmint tea or cool rosemary tea.
- Ulcers require stronger therapy; infusions containing chamomile, fennel, lemon balm and marshmallow are particularly beneficial. Fennel is an excellent pain reliever, especially after a meal and can be combined with American cranesbill. Your local health food shop will be able to order this for you. Chamomile reduces the spasm around the ulcer and marshmallow leaves cut down excess acid production in the stomach.

ACUPUNCTURE

This is one of the most effective complimentary therapies for healing stomach ulcers. Once you realise that needles are virtually painless, it can be quite relaxing. As it requires several visits to an acupuncturist, which can be expensive, I tend to reserve it for the more severe cases. Nevertheless, a great number of people have derived tremendous relief, after only two or three sessions. For more information on acupuncture, please refer back to Chapter 3.

The principle of treatment is to 'pacify' the stomach using a combination of local and distal points. The needles are left in place for about thirty minutes, with either intermittent stimulation by hand, or continous stimulation by an electrical pulsar. The particular points where the needles are placed are Stomach 36 and Ren 12 (see Figure 5.2) which pacify the stomach and relieve pain. Liver 13 and Stomach 44 promote digestion and relieve stomach fullness and Pericardium 6 stops nausea and vomiting. For the relevant earpoint, turn to Figure 3.2 on page 20. Heat (moxibustion) applied to the end of the needles will increase the effect of the acupuncture by further stimulating the flow of *Chi* through the appropriate channel.

Christine had experienced very severe abdominal pain, which was associated with food, over a period of only four weeks. An endoscopy had revealed a large ulcer, about the size of a fifty pence piece, at the outlet of her stomach. So far the ulcer had not been healed by conventional drugs. She was still in agony and was virtually unable to eat.

Acupuncture can produce almost instant results. When I started Christine's first session she was in agony, but within five minutes of the needles being stimulated, her pain had virtually disappeared. When the needles were removed, however, the pain returned though not as severe. Nevertheless, Christine was convinced that acupuncture was likely to work for her in the long term.

I treated her three times a week, for three weeks, and then weekly for a further month. During that time, her pain subsided. Now she only has the occasional twinge. Christine comes to see me for a reinforcing session, once a month, although I will hopefully be able to reduce these very soon. Although I did not advise her to, she stopped conventional treatment when the acupuncture began, so it is fairly certain that it produced her recovery.

Conclusion

From both the doctor's and patient's viewpoint, the treatment of indigestion and stomach ulcers with acupuncture is the most effective as relief of the severest symptoms can be achieved with relative ease. It is a

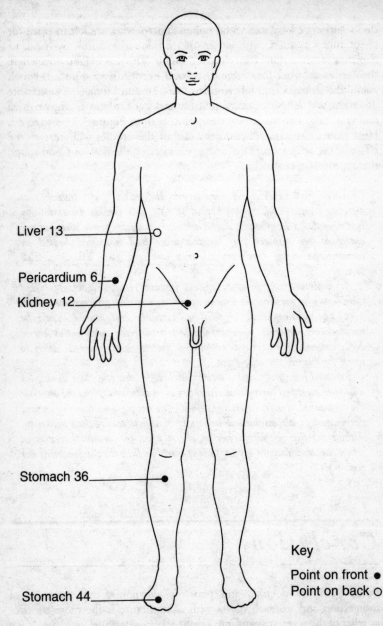

Liver 13

Pericardium 6

Kidney 12

Stomach 36

Stomach 44

Key

Point on front ●
Point on back ○

Figure 5.2 Acupuncture points for indigestion and ulceration

classic situation where orthodox and alternative medicine come together, to produce a cure.

A vast array of different treatments are available for both indigestion and ulcers. During my years in practice, I have found the methods described in this chapter the simplest to follow, and the most successful. To help you, they are summarised in the plan below.

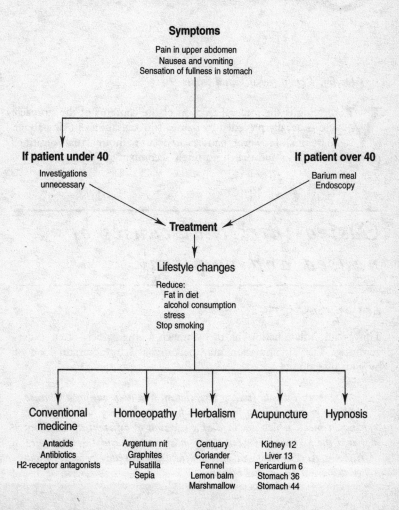

TREATMENT PLAN FOR INDIGESTION AND STOMACH ULCERS

Symptoms

Pain in upper abdomen
Nausea and vomiting
Sensation of fullness in stomach

If patient under 40

Investigations
unnecessary

If patient over 40

Barium meal
Endoscopy

Treatment

Lifestyle changes

Reduce:
  Fat in diet
  alcohol consumption
  stress
Stop smoking

Conventional medicine	Homoeopathy	Herbalism	Acupuncture	Hypnosis
Antacids	Argentum nit	Centaury	Kidney 12	
Antibiotics	Graphites	Coriander	Liver 13	
H2-receptor antagonists	Pulsatilla	Fennel	Pericardium 6	
	Sepia	Lemon balm	Stomach 36	
		Marshmallow	Stomach 44	

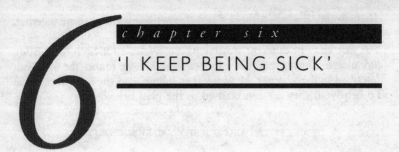

chapter six

'1 KEEP BEING SICK'

‹ *Doctor, I often feel sick and vomit.* ›

Vomiting is the forceful ejection of the contents of the stomach and is usually preceded by nausea (the sensation of being about to be sick). However, nausea can occur without actual vomiting. Increased salivation and diarrhoea often accompany vomiting.

Gastro-intestinal causes of nausea and vomiting

ACUTE GASTRITIS

This is an inflammation of the stomach lining which often causes vomiting. The inflammation may be provoked by a certain food or by viral infection.

> *Twenty seven year old Julie, a receptionist, had been out for a Chinese meal one evening with a few friends from work. They had chosen the banquet menu which consisted of a selection of different dishes. They shared the following between them: meat, seafood and all served with fried rice. As it was a special occasion Julie had travelled by taxi to allow her to have a few glasses of wine.*

Sometime during the night, however, Julie was woken by a rumbling in her stomach and a feeling of intense nausea. Julie was sick several times during the night, so by the time I visited her, just before morning surgery, she looked terrible. She suspected food poisoning and vowed never to go to that restaurant again! In fact, her condition was not due to food poisoning (see following section).

On examination, the upper part of Julie's abdomen felt mildly tender but there were no other abnormalities. She was simply suffering from the effects of eating far too much of the wrong sort of food. Most stomachs cannot take a sudden increase in quantity or a change in the type of food eaten. Julie never eats seafood and rarely drinks so much wine, so her stomach did not know what had hit it!

FOOD POISONING

Food poisoning (a form of gastro-enteritis) can cause intense vomiting and is less common than acute gastritis. It may be caused by certain types of food, by bacterial or viral infection.

Ray, a businessman, had been away at a conference. Dinner on the last night had been held at a nearby country club. The alternatives on the menu were chicken or salmon, and about six hours after the meal finished, most of the guests who had eaten the chicken developed persistent vomiting. This was accompanied by intense diarrhoea, which indicated it was acute gastro-enteritis, rather than acute gastritis. When public health officials were called in, it was found the chicken had been infected with the bacteria called Salmonella, probably because it had been cooked for too short a time, or because it had been re-heated. Ray slowly recovered but it took ten days for his symptoms to settle whereas Julie, with simple gastritis, was back at work after forty eight hours.

STOMACH ULCER

Nausea and vomiting may be the only symptoms of a stomach ulcer, although intense pain usually accompanies the sickness. Vomiting due to an ulcer usually relieves the pain. The previous chapter (Chapter 5) deals with this condition.

Some medications can cause vomiting. These include antibiotics such as erythromycin, co-trimoxazole and tetracycline; digoxin, various analgesics including co-proxamol and some anti-depressants. The most common drug, however, is aspirin.

Every time you take an aspirin tablet, it causes slight irritation of the stomach lining (less likely if you take them in water). It is fine to take a full strength tablet occasionally to relieve headaches but prolonged and regular use of aspirin can be very damaging to the stomach.

MEDICINES

Fifty nine year old Nora had read, in one of the women's magazines, that aspirin aids the circulation and reduces the risk of heart disease and strokes. Unfortunately, this magazine did not mention in which cases this was appropriate, give the recommended dose nor did it warn of any possible side-effects. Nora bought some aspirin from the local supermarket and took two twice daily. The tablets she was taking contained 300 mg of aspirin so her total daily dose was 1200 mg. A daily dose of 75 mg dissolved in water is sufficient to boost the circulation. Nora was, therefore, taking fifteen times the recommended dose! Eventually her stomach became so inflamed, that she started to vomit.

ALCOHOL

One particular drug that commonly causes vomiting – alcohol. While many of us drink small amounts socially (indeed, this may actually be of benefit to our health), it is very toxic in large quantities. Anyone who finds themselves persistently vomiting the morning after, is obviously doing no good to their digestive system and may well be on their way to alcoholism.

Geoff had a history of being sick after breakfast on most days. The vomit was small in quantity and contained mucus, sometimes with flecks of blood. He commented that he often experienced 'dry heaves', usually when cleaning his teeth. This latter symptom occurs commonly in alcoholics. Geoff did not realise that, by volunteering this information, he was virtually giving me the diagnosis. On direct questioning, he became quite aggressive and flatly denied any alcohol problem, so there was little I could do to convince him. However, some time after he left the surgery, his wife phoned to say that she had in fact persuaded him to come and see me about his drinking, because he was consuming about three to four bottles of whisky per day.

GALL STONES

Bile is produced by the liver and stored in the gall bladder and if it becomes too concentrated then gall stones can form. If a stone becomes stuck at the outlet of the gall bladder then vomiting may occur. However, it is accompanied by severe, right-sided, abdominal pain just below the rib cage so there is little doubt about the diagnosis. I have dealt with gall stones in Chapter 9.

OBSTRUCTION

If a blockage occurs anywhere along the digestive system then vomiting can occur. This blockage is known as intestinal obstruction, which is caused by a variety of factors including twisted bowel and diverticulitis (see Chapter 13). The symptoms of obstruction are vomiting, pain and abdominal distension. Usually, hospital admission is required to correct fluid loss. Once this has been achieved, an operation may be needed to relieve the obstruction.

If the outlet of the stomach is blocked, then persistent vomiting occurs in large volume, accompanied by rapid weight loss. The cause of this may be a large stomach ulcer. In rare cases, it may also be due to cancer.

CONSTIPATION

If constipation is severe, then it may act as a dam, blocking undigested food. Eventually, the blockage may be so severe that vomiting results. (For more information on this condition, please see Chapter 10.)

APPENDICITIS

The appendix is a small tube attached to the caecum (the chamber which links the small and large intestines; see diagram on page 7). Occasionally it becomes blocked and infection results. The main symptom is severe, low, right-sided abdominal pain. Vomiting and nausea may often accompany the pain. I have dealt with this more fully in Chapter 15. Appendicitis must be treated as an emergency and requires immediate hospital treatment.

Non-digestive causes of nausea and vomiting

The automatic reaction of everyone who feels sick is to think there is something wrong with their stomach. However, this is not always the case. Other causes are listed below.

PREGNANCY

Nausea and vomiting are symptoms associated with the first trimester of pregnancy. These usually disappear by the beginning or middle of the second trimester. It typically occurs in the early morning but can also start in the afternoon or evening. The condition is rarely serious, but can be distressing.

THYROID DISORDERS

The thyroid is a large gland situated in the front of the neck controlling the rate at which the body functions. Both an underactive and an overactive thyroid gland can result in vomiting but this will be associated with other symptoms. Overactivity causes diarrhoea, breathlessness, weight loss and a fast heart rate; an underactive gland gives constipation, thick, dry skin and extreme fatigue.

MIGRAINE

Vomiting may be a prominent feature of migraine. The characteristic, one-sided headache, which feels as though it is boring through an eye and may be associated with flashing lights, usually makes the diagnosis certain. A minority of patients suffer abdominal pain with migraine and this can lead to needless investigation of the digestive system.

MIDDLE EAR DISEASE

As well as allowing us to hear, the ear also controls our balance. When this mechanism becomes disturbed, either by infection or by a circulatory disturbance, then vomiting occurs. It is accompanied by extreme dizziness and vomiting only occurs when the head is moved.

MENSTRUATION

A small proportion of women suffer from vomiting at a certain stage in their menstrual cycle. It is thought that the hormone, oestrogen, affects the muscular co-ordination of the stomach.

ANOREXIA NERVOSA

This is a complicated disorder which some doctors would class solely as psychological. However, it is worth mentioning it here because of the drastic effects it can have on the digestive system.

Anna, a twenty four year old woman, came to see me because of persistent vomiting. She hadn't really wanted to consult a doctor but her husband was very concerned about her. She denied any weight loss and said she thought she was too heavy. Her husband mentioned that Anna was now much thinner than when they had married, two years ago. On examination, her bones were easily visible, the upper part of her abdomen was very tender and the lower part was distended with retained wind. When the abdomen distends in this way it is usually from a dietary problem: eating too much, too little or the wrong sort of food. I was certain that Anna was hardly eating anything although she still saw herself as too fat.

Sufferers of Anorexia nervosa typically have a distorted view of their body. They feel that the vomiting is an effective means of preventing the food they eat being absorbed thus stopping any weight gain. Management of the condition is very difficult as it hinges on convincing the patient to accept a more normal view of her body image and a balanced view of food. However, patients with this condition, are reluctant to take any advice. They usually need psychiatric help, and Anna agreed to be referred. I prescribed the homoeopathic remedy, Argentum nit, which can be useful in stimulating the appetite while waiting for the hospital appointment.

BULIMIA NERVOSA

This eating disorder can be differentiated from anorexia in that it is characterised by bouts of serious overeating, followed by copious, self-induced vomiting, which is provoked by guilt. It produces gross abdominal distension and, unlike anorexia, weight loss is not a significant feature. Again, referral for psychiatric treatment is needed.

Periodic vomiting

About twenty per cent of the people I see in the surgery who complain of sickness can find no obvious reason for their vomiting. It is extremely frustrating for both patient and doctor who are obviously both keen to identify a cause. The attacks of vomiting are usually brief and patients do not seek advice until several episodes have occurred.

Undoubtedly, there is still a great deal we do not understand about the workings of the human body. I am in fact convinced that nausea and vomiting of this kind must indicate an underlying problem in the stomach which has not yet been discovered. I have therefore, included it in this section of the book. I refer to unexplained sickness of this kind as periodic vomiting. Doctors who believe it to be a psychological problem refer to it as psychogenic vomiting.

There is no doubt that stress is closely linked with periodic vomiting and this is perhaps why many specialists think it is a nervous disorder. However, the exact reason why stress should produce sickness is, as yet, unknown. Stress affects individuals in different ways. It almost seems to pick out a weakness in our bodies. Some people will therefore have headaches, others skin problems, palpitations or experience frequent urination. This does not mean that we are mentally ill, simply that this is the particular way in which stress affects us.

When vomiting is due to stress, there are no other features of organic disease and very rarely is there significant fluid loss or dehydration. The stress and any accompanying anxiety are often relieved by the vomiting. It is almost as if the sickness works as a safety valve. In children cyclical vomiting (often occuring each day) can be the result of domestic tensions or problems at school.

SUMMARY OF CAUSES OF NAUSEA AND VOMITING

Gastro-intestinal	**Non-digestive**	**Periodic vomiting**
Acute gastritis	Pregnancy	
Stomach ulcer	Hormone imbalance	
Intestinal obstruction	Thyroid disorders	
Constipation	Migraine	
Stomach cancer (rare)	Middle ear disease	
Drugs	Anorexia nervosa	
Gall stones	Bulimia nervosa	
Appendicitis		

Investigations

If the reason for the vomiting is very obvious then no investigations are needed. Morning sickness during the early stages of pregnancy is also easily recognised. Disorders such as hormone imbalance or thyroid disease can be shown by a simple blood test. Migraine is apparent from the patient's history. Middle ear disease is associated with dizziness on moving the head, whilst anorexia and bulimia are both evident from the person's appearance.

However, where the cause is not easily identifiable, then routine investigations should be carried out.

BLOOD TESTS

It is important to test the blood routinely as anaemia can be indicative of microscopic bleeding from the stomach, which is often a feature of stomach ulcers and malignant tumours. If vomiting is severe, then the concentration of urea (waste products) in the blood may be elevated, indicating dehydration. Where intestinal obstruction has occurred the disturbance of body chemicals can be so severe, that the whole balance of chemicals in the blood is upset.

BARIUM MEAL

The swallowing of barium sulphate followed by a series of X-ray pictures, will clearly show any mechanical abnormality in the stomach, including ulcers and malignant tumours.

ENDOSCOPY

This is, without doubt, the most accurate investigation of all, which allows the inside of the stomach to be viewed directly. A flexible fibre-optic tube is passed into the stomach, which has a light at the bottom end and an eyepiece at the other. Thanks to this investigation, the specialist can easily identify gastritis, erosions caused by certain drugs, ulcers, growths and any blockages.

ULTRASOUND SCAN

This gives a much clearer picture of the inside of the abdomen and is non-invasive. Sound waves are emitted by a device called a transducer and are echoed by the organs and tissues of the body. The transducer picks up these echoes which are then translated into a two-dimensional image on a screen. This is particularly useful in identifying gall stones.

At the age of forty seven, Jim had developed a tendency to vomit every morning after breakfast. He joked that he didn't think he was pregnant! He tended to have some pain in his upper abdomen before being sick, but this was relieved by the vomiting. His diet was reasonably healthy – he ate plenty of wholefoods and didn't suffer from heartburn or indigestion. He slept well and never woke up with stomach pains. More recently the sickness had also occurred when he came in from work and he thought his weight had dropped by about half a stone. Jim's bowel function was regular.

On examination, his stomach was soft, had no areas of tenderness and was not distended. All his other systems were healthy and there was no sign of metabolic disease.

This vomiting did not seem to fit any condition perfectly. It could be simple gastritis, triggered by breakfast, but the sickness did not occur after other meals. A low grade stomach ulcer was another possibility, but he was not experiencing the characteristic symptoms: extreme pain, waking up at night and abdominal tenderness. It was obvious he did not have an acute intestinal obstruction as his abdomen was not distended and the pain was neither severe enough or in the right place for gall stones. He looked too well to have cancer (usually there is loss of appetite and considerable weight loss). He said he had not been taking aspirin or any other medication.

In summary, he had one or two features of all the digestive disorders that can cause vomiting, but nothing to clinch the diagnosis.

I advised Jim to have investigations (listed above) over the next month and all were normal, apart from a mild inflammation revealed by the endoscopy, which was suggestive of a low-grade gastritis. I did not think, however, that this would be sufficient to cause Jim's symptoms and suspected stress also had a part to play. I discovered that Jim was manager of a local bank and he had become very worried about the possibility of redundancy. As most banks now seem to recruit younger people, Jim was concerned that if he were sacked, then there would be little prospect of further work. The onset of his vomiting had coincided with all this tension, so it was reasonable to assume, that the sickness was due to low-grade gastritis and high stress levels. This assumption was supported by the test results, which were normal.

Conventional treatment

⟨ Look doctor, can't you just give me something to stop the sickness? ⟩

This is all too common a reaction these days – people simply want to swallow a tablet, without attempting to search for the cause of their disorder.

Drugs can be beneficial in the treatment of symptoms while the cause of the disorder is under investigation. Routine usage should be avoided. However, if a patient refuses investigations, then a doctor must respect their decision.

The type of drug prescribed depends to some extent on the possible cause of the upset. Antihistamines, for example, are particularly useful for the treatment of middle ear disturbances and travel sickness. However, such drugs have little use in vomiting from a gastro-intestinal cause.

Metoclopramide or Domperidone are the conventional drugs which are prescribed most often. They are highly effective antiemetics (drugs which prevent vomiting). Not only do they inhibit the vomiting reflex, but they also make vomiting far less likely by speeding up the passage of food through the stomach.

I prefer to prescribe Domperidone as one per cent of patients taking Metoclopramide experience side-effects, (mainly loss of co-ordination).

There are only three situations where a conventional antiemetic is of value:

- If the vomiting is from an acute infection or irritation of the stomach, as in food induced or viral gastritis;
- If nausea and vomiting are due to drugs (such as digoxin which is used in the treatment of heart conditions) this situation can be extremely difficult to treat. If use of such drugs is essential, combining it with an antiemetic may still allow the medication to be used;
- If the patient is undergoing chemotherapy (used in the treatment of cancer). As this can produce severe nausea and vomiting, antiemetics can be vital.

Nausea and vomiting in the first trimester of pregnancy does not usually require drug therapy. As there is a risk of damage to the baby, any conventional medication should be reserved for very severe cases where there is a danger to the mother. I use either homoeopathic remedies, usually Nux vomica, or acupuncture which carry no risk to mother or baby (see pages 63–65).

Alternative treatment

SELF-HELP

If you have vomited or feel nauseous, it is advisable to maintain your fluid intake and avoid dairy products. As the vomiting subsides, a light diet can be introduced. The first solid food should be plain, toasted, wholemeal bread and a little clear vegetable soup. If these are tolerated, the next step is plain boiled, brown rice with some steamed vegetables (carrots are particularly recommended). Finally, a normal diet can be reintroduced over the next couple of days.

COUNSELLING

Where stress is a major contributing factor, counselling can be very effective. This gives the patient the opportunity to talk through a problem with someone who is trained to guide the conversation in a helpful direction. A counsellor's views are not biased in any way. All meetings with a counsellor are entirely confidential, even from your doctor, enabling the patient to be much more open about their problems. Any notes are taken to help refresh the counsellor's memory in subsequent meetings and do not contain prejudicial information.

Although it was impossible to prove that tension at work had caused his vomiting, Jim's sickness had started after the threat of redundancy. It was important for him to cope with the stress he was under, so I referred him to our practice counsellor. Jim had a course of six sessions during which he was able to talk through his dilemma and find ways in which he could modify his response to stress. The counsellor taught him some relaxation techniques and lent him a relaxation tape for use at home. In just six weeks, Jim felt a great deal better in himself, although his physical symptoms were still very much the same.

HOMOEOPATHY

I find it is necessary in cases such as these to combine two, maybe three, types of natural therapy to produce a cure. This is logical as they each stimulate different parts of our natural healing process. Homoeopathy is often the most effective way of controlling vomiting.

As always, the choice of homoeopathic remedy depends on the lifestyle and personality of the individual, as well as their symptoms (in Jim's case vomiting). When sickness occurs the appropriate homoeopathic tablets should be taken every fifteen minutes, until the vomiting stops. These tablets have the great advantage of dissolving under the tongue rather than in the stomach so cannot themselves cause stomach irritation.

If you simply buy the first homoeopathic remedy you see, you may not pick the right one. You may then be tempted to say that homoeopathy doesn't work for you. It is therefore important to choose a remedy which suits your own features.

Pulsatilla

Pulsatilla (which comes from the Windflower) is recommended for fair haired people, who often have blue eyes and a pale complexion (usually with some pink patches). They are affectionate, easily moved to tears or laughter, shy never obstinate, but like and indeed seek sympathy. Such people are also sensitive to reprimand, tend to put on fat easily and dislike extremes in weather.

Pulsatilla is effective in the treatment of vomiting which comes on after food and which is worse in the morning and evening. You may also find that the nausea improves in the open air, with cold compresses or after taking cold food and drinks.

Nux vomica

Perhaps the most widely used of all the homoeopathic remedies for sickness. It can be used for vomiting which occurs two to three hours after eating and where retching is painful. There may also be a tendency to wake around four in the morning and an inability to return to sleep. In addition, the sufferer may feel hungover – especially after a heavy meal or rich food. It is a remedy suitable for thin, dark people who are inclined to be impatient and irritable. They typically lead a sedentary life and are hypersensitive to noise, light and smell. They are most comfortable in a warm environment, when alone and in the rain.

Ipecac

This is the best remedy for persistent nausea and griping pains in the stomach. The vomit may contain green mucus and is associated with headache and perspiration. Lying down also increases the feeling of nausea. This particular remedy is suitable for easy-going, relaxed people who are very open with their feelings. Such people often suffer from travel sickness.

Arsenicum album

This remedy is suited to excessively tidy, intelligent and precise individuals, who like cold, windy weather. Perversely, the pain they experience in their stomachs improves when heat is applied. When the vomiting occurs their reaction may be out of proportion with their condition and is often accompanied by irritability. The stomach pains are of a burning nature and the sickness is preceded by a period of intense nausea.

Pulsatilla was the best choice of remedy for Jim, as it was suited to his personality and physical features. After a few day's treatment, the vomiting episodes cleared.

HERBAL MEDICINE

Chamomile

Sometimes patients ask me to give them something which will really soothe the stomach.

Chamomile was called 'ground apple' by the ancient Greeks because of its smell. As the flower is the most potent part of the herb, herbalists developed double-flowered varieties to increase the yield from each plant. Commercial tea bags are now widely available but you may find the taste rather watery and insipid. A single flower, dried at home, gives much more flavour and appears to be a good deal more effective.

Ginger

If you do not like the taste of chamomile tea, then ginger is a suitable alternative. It was originally brought in from tropical Asia and has been used as a medicinal herb in the West for over 2000 years. A hot, dry herb, ginger was traditionally used to warm the stomach and dispel chills. In the eighteenth century it was added to many remedies to reduce the irritant effects they may have on the stomach.

For nausea and vomiting, the root is the vital part and it is best taken as a tincture (a solution in alcohol) which is available from health food stores. Another option is crystallised ginger, which can be chewed whenever required.

Cloves
The latin name of this herb is *Syzygium aromaticum*. It can be taken as an infusion. The simplest way, however, is to take one to two drops of the essential oil on a sugar lump. Although it can be extremely effective, its strong flavour can sometimes limit its use.

ACUPUNCTURE

This form of therapy is particularly effective in cases of persistent nausea and vomiting. But it means seeing a therapist which can be time consuming and expensive, so I am cautious when recommending it. However, there is a single acupuncture point on the foot which, if massaged with the end of a finger, can bring instant relief. This is the point called Liver 3 (see diagram below). It can also be useful for other types of vomiting, including pregnancy sickness.

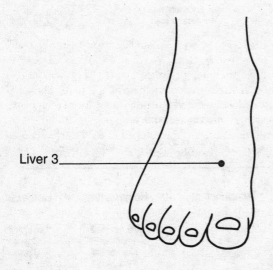

Liver 3

Figure 6.1   Acupuncture point for Nausea and Vomiting

TREATMENT PLAN FOR NAUSEA AND VOMITING

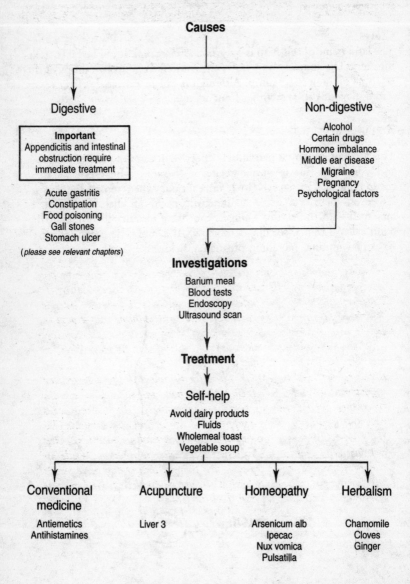

Causes

Digestive

> **Important**
> Appendicitis and intestinal
> obstruction require
> immediate treatment

Acute gastritis
Constipation
Food poisoning
Gall stones
Stomach ulcer

(*please see relevant chapters*)

Non-digestive

Alcohol
Certain drugs
Hormone imbalance
Middle ear disease
Migraine
Pregnancy
Psychological factors

Investigations

Barium meal
Blood tests
Endoscopy
Ultrasound scan

Treatment

Self-help

Avoid dairy products
Fluids
Wholemeal toast
Vegetable soup

Conventional medicine

Antiemetics
Antihistamines

Acupuncture

Liver 3

Homeopathy

Arsenicum alb
Ipecac
Nux vomica
Pulsatilla

Herbalism

Chamomile
Cloves
Ginger

7 REACTIONS TO FOOD

*O*ne morning John, a twenty two year old man, ate a biscuit with his morning coffee. Within a few minutes, he collapsed and was desperately short of breath. One of his workmates realised there was no time to wait for an ambulance and drove him to the surgery.

When I examined him, he was virtually unconscious: he had stopped breathing and his blood pressure was so low that it did not register on the recording machine. His face was swollen and his skin was blotchy. It appeared that John had suffered acute anaphylaxis (a severe allergic reaction). An injection of adrenalin and antihistamine into a vein in John's arm, quickly restored his normal blood pressure and breathing.

When he regained consciousness, he told me that he was allergic to nuts but hadn't realised that the biscuit he had eaten had contained them. Closer examination of the packet indicated that one of the ingredients was almond essence. John now takes extra care with everything he eats but, in case he unknowingly eats anything with nuts in it, he always carries a supply of adrenalin around with him. This is a pre-packed syringe containing 1 ml of adrenalin which is injected just below the skin at the first sign of an allergic reaction. While an allergy of this severity is very rare, it is thought that one in three people suffer abnormal reactions to food. These can be divided into the separate categories of food allergies and food intolerance.

Allergy

Allergies have recently come to the fore of public attention. Certain elements in food have been linked to a wide range of symptoms, some of which are gastro-intestinal. The immune system forms antibodies when it recognises harmful substances (antigens). When someone is allergic, their immune system responds to a particular substance which may not provoke any reaction in other people (hay fever is a common example). The exact reason for this remains unclear.

The concept of food allergy was first introduced in the United States but was slow to cross the Atlantic. Scepticism has grown because, as food allergy became popular, some self-styled allergy therapists claimed that virtually any disease could be caused by food. However, there is no doubt the condition exists and it is probably underdiagnosed in this country.

The symptoms of food allergy are usually mild, but very annoying. An itchy rash, swelling around the eyes plus diarrhoea and vomiting is the usual presentation.

COMMON FOOD ALLERGY SYMPTOMS

| **Extreme** | Asphyxia | **Topical** (**affecting the skin**) | Wheals Swelling Eczema |
| **Digestive** | Vomiting Abdominal pain Distension Diarrhoea | **Respiratory** | Runny nose Wheezing Sneezing |

The list of potential allergens is a long one but the most common are citrus fruits, eggs, cheese, cow's milk, nuts, wheat, yeast, beans and pulses. Certain additives such as tartrazine (B102), benzoates (E210–219) and metabisulphate are also allergens and are present in many soft drinks and sweets. These additives frequently provoke reactions in children, typically an itchy rash around the mouth from saliva which has mixed with the allergen. Hyperactivity has also been linked to food allergies, particularly with artificial additives.

In some cases, the cause is more obscure. Jason, a nine year old boy, came to the surgery with persistent allergic rashes and swelling around the eyes. It seemed to be related to food or drink, but all the allergy tests he had undergone at the hospital were negative. This situation went on for a year until, one day, I visited his brother who was ill in bed with measles. It was the first time I had been to their house, as Jason always came into the surgery. Until then, I had not been aware that it was at the bottom of a country lane. Isolated houses often do not have their water pipes maintained, so I sent a sample of the drinking water to the pathology lab. Analysis revealed a high level of copper. As soon as Jason switched to bottled water his allergy settled, and he has never had any problems of this nature since.

Intolerance

This occurs when certain foodstuffs cause an irritation to the digestive system. As symptoms predominantly occur in the gut, food intolerance can be differentiated from food allergy (which triggers a generalised body reaction leading to all kinds of symptoms, not just those of a gastro-intestinal nature).

The symptoms of food intolerance come on much more slowly than those of food allergies (up to forty eight hours after eating). The exact reason for food intolerance is not known, but it probably arises, either from a direct effect of a certain food on the intestine lining, or from some defect in the structure of the wall of the gut.

Food allergies are triggered by a minute amount of the offending foodstuff. In contrast, food intolerance, is generally caused by an excessive amount of the particular food or its reintroduction to the diet, after a period of absence. Regular ingestion of small amounts may only provoke minor gut reactions or, in some cases, a feeling of fatigue. Experts believe this is because your body's defence mechanism has the ability to deal with small quantities of the irritant food, but this mechanism breaks down when challenged with larger amounts.

Any food can be implicated, although a reaction to milk is perhaps the most common. Milk contains a sugar called lactose which some people cannot tolerate. A more serious condition is a sensitivity to gluten which produces a condition called coeliac disease (dealt with in Chapter 8).

Twenty eight year old Carol presented me with a tricky problem: she was complaining of intermittent abdominal pains and occasional vomiting. She felt generally rather lethargic, but not specifically ill. As full examination and routine tests did not reveal any abnormality, I began to suspect food intolerance. Trying to find the cause, however, was difficult. Excluding milk and wheat from the diet made no difference.

Carol would suffer these digestive symptoms about three days a week, which certainly affected her quality of life. Then, one Saturday night, she went out for a meal with some friends and had a beautiful piece of poached salmon. The following day, the abdominal pain was much worse and she was sick several times. In hindsight, the cause was obvious: Carol had not eaten salmon before then but she did have fish paste in her sandwiches for lunch, three days a week. Omitting the paste cured her symptoms.

Management

The most effective treatment for both allergy and intolerance is a diet which avoids the food causing the symptoms. If the cause of the allergy or intolerance is obvious, then the cure is simple. However, isolating the offending foodstuff may not always be a straightforward procedure.

Mark was suffering with persistent stomach pains and an itchy rash, which seemed to worsen after eating. He had absolutely no idea which food could be causing the reaction. This was a few years ago, when the vogue was to eat only one type of meat or fruit, and only drink spring water for a week. When the symptoms had subsided completely, various foods were reintroduced, one at a time, while watching for those that provoked the reaction. Pears were thought to contain very few allergens, so Mark went away with instructions for a week's diet of pears and spring water!

Not surprisingly, when he returned his symptoms were no different, mainly because an elimination diet is more easily said, than done. Mark only managed a day and a half of eating pear after pear, before he cracked and turned to more nourishing food. In fact, the flatulence caused by eating so many pears was far more uncomfortable than his original symptoms!

I have now stopped using a diet anything like as strict as this as it is both too difficult and too unpleasant for anyone to take for a long enough time. Analysis of the foods which provoke symptoms in over ninety per cent of my patients, during the last five years, has allowed me, in consultation with the more effective dietician at our practice, to develop an elimination diet. It is possible that the foods allowed by the exclusion diet may still provoke the symptoms but if patients keep to the diet and record the timing of all foods eaten in relation to symptoms, then it is possible to spot the offenders quite easily. Rather than make a long list of the foods that must be eliminated, the following chart indicates the only foods which are allowed.

EXCLUSION DIET
White fish
All meat (except sausages, bacon and preserved meats)
All vegetables except potatoes and onions
Apples, bananas and pears
Rice, Rice Krispies
Sunflower oil, olive oil
Goats' milk, soya milk
Herbal tea
Fresh apple, pineapple and tomato juices
Salt, herbs and sugar

After two weeks on the exclusion diet, when all the symptoms have cleared, the excluded foods are reintroduced, one at a time. Those that do not cause problems, are added to the basic diet. When all testing is finished, then the diet is checked for nutritional adequacy. Often supplements of iron, calcium and vitamin C are advisable.

Occasionally, some patients will not stick to the diet and treatment of the symptoms may be needed. A technique is currently being developed, where it is possible to desensitise the patient, by putting very dilute quantities of the offending foodstuff under the tongue. This is only in the early stages of development, but nevertheless looks promising.

TREATMENT PLAN FOR FOOD ALLERGY AND INTOLERANCE

**Symptoms peculiar
to allergy**

Asphyxia
Rash
Runny nose
Sneezing
Swelling
Wheezing

**Symptoms shared by both
allergy and intolerance**

Diarrhoea
Distension of abdomen
Pain in abdomen
Vomiting

**Identifiable
cause**

**No apparent
cause**

Exclusion diet

Omit allergen from diet

Treatment of symptoms

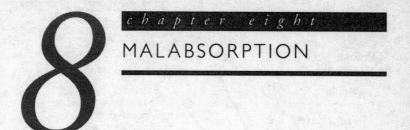

chapter eight

MALABSORPTION

I n some people, the complex process of digestion (described fully in Chapter 2) is impaired. The food which is eaten fails to be absorbed and therefore does not provide adequate nutrition. This condition is known as malabsorption syndrome. There are two main causes: inadequate digestion of food and diseases of the small intestine.

Inadequate digestion of food

In this situation food is not in the correct state to be absorbed when it reaches the ileum, as a result of the following reasons.

STOMACH SURGERY

Twenty years ago, the only effective treatment for stomach ulcers was to remove the part of the stomach which produces acid (approximately one third of its capacity). This leads to inadequate mixing of food with digestive juices in the stomach and rapid stomach emptying. In normal circumstances, when food leaves the stomach, it triggers the release of enzymes by the pancreas. This reflex is lost after surgery, further inhibiting digestion. Increasing weakness and fatigue are common symptoms. Blood tests may often indicate anaemia as a result of malabsorption of iron.

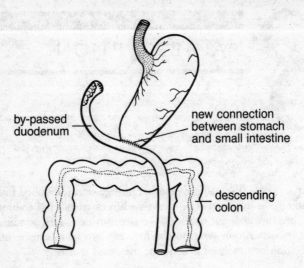

by-passed
duodenum

new connection
between stomach
and small intestine

descending
colon

Figure 8.1   Impaired digestion after stomach surgery

INSUFFICIENT PRODUCTION
OF PANCREATIC ENZYMES

The pancreas gland sits in the loop of the duodenum, and produces
several enzymes. If the pancreas becomes inflamed or infected, a
condition called pancreatitis develops. This inhibits the production of
enzymes, resulting in malabsorption.

Diseases of the small intestine

Damage to the lining of the duodenum and ileum, will cause malabsorption by reducing the surface area which can absorb digested food. Earlier
this century, the main cause of destruction of the ileum's surface was
tuberculosis. Happily, this is now rare. Today, the two significant
conditions are intolerance of cow's milk and coeliac disease.

INTOLERANCE OF COW'S MILK

This condition is quite common in babies where the lining of the intestine is not fully developed and until it does, cow's milk cannot be absorbed.

Jamie, a five week old baby, had developed severe diarrhoea and was obviously losing weight. At birth, he was a healthy eight pounds, nine ounces but, at five weeks, weighed only just over seven pounds. Initially, he had fed very well but now his mother was struggling with every bottle. Jamie was fed on one brand of dried milk but changing brands did not produce any improvement.

On examination, Jamie looked thin and had that worried look that babies show when they have lost weight. Otherwise I could find nothing abnormal. I was sure intolerance of cow's milk was Jamie's problem and as soon as he switched to soya milk, he rapidly gained weight.

COELIAC DISEASE

This condition seems to affect far greater numbers of people in the West, compared to Africa or Asia. In my own practice, several patients in a wide age group have had this disorder, so it is worth considering in some detail.

The disease is caused by a sensitivity to gluten (a protein present in wheat and rye flour). The range of foods which contains this is surprisingly wide. In some way, gluten is toxic to the lining of the small intestine, destroying the villi, eventually causing malabsorption (there is insufficient surface area left to absorb the food).

Clinical features
The symptoms usually begin, either in the first three years of life or in early adulthood. The child ceases to thrive and is irritable and fractious. The fat content in the stools increases becoming loose, very pale, bulky and offensive-smelling. The stools float on water and are difficult to flush away.

In a child, the diagnosis is clear from the colour of the stools and the failure to gain weight. In adults, however, diagnosis is more complicated as symptoms can include mild anaemia and listlessness, due to malabsorption of iron and folic acid. Malabsorption, diarrhoea, steatorrhoea (offensive-smelling stools), severe anaemia and marked weight loss may also occur.

The following three cases illustrate the extent to which the symptoms of coeliac disease can vary.

Jackie, *a twenty year old secretary, came to my surgery with a five day history of headache, sore throat and general malaise. It appeared to be a simple infection and I reassured her she would feel better in a few days. Two weeks later, Jackie returned with diarrhoea (her stools were loose, pale and smelt very offensive). These features were strongly suggestive of malabsorption and a duodenal biopsy supported the diagnosis of coeliac disease.*

Once Jackie began a gluten-free diet, her symptoms quickly settled. After six months, a repeat biopsy showed improvement in the lining of the intestine, with the villi growing back to normal.

Unfortunately Jackie did not have much faith in the diagnosis, mainly because she didn't like the idea of being on the diet for life. She, therefore, returned to her usual diet for the following three months. Diarrhoea and pale stools soon returned, and a further biopsy showed renewed villus damage. At this stage, Jackie realised she would need to be on a life-long gluten-free diet, and she has had no further problems.

Margaret, *a fifty three year old part-time clerical officer, came to the surgery because her skin had lost all its colour. She had also developed a huge cold sore on her lower lip which she, quite understandably, felt was unsightly and embarrassing.*

On examination, Margaret looked grossly anaemic. This was proved by a blood test which showed her haemoglobin was only 4.6 gm. The level of haemoglobin (the iron-containing protein which transports oxygen in the blood) should normally be over 12 gm. Margaret's level was a third of the normal amount.

She was sent to hospital, as a level this low necessitates blood transfusion. During her stay there, no obvious cause for her anaemia was found, until a duodenal biopsy showed changes typical of coeliac disease. Although the lining of the small intestine was grossly abnormal, at no time did Margaret develop any diarrhoea or steatorrhoea. Medicine is rarely a simple science!

Tina, *a twenty one year old student nurse, came into the surgery with general malaise, abdominal bloating and mild diarrhoea. As early as seventeen months old, she had experienced the typical features of childhood coeliac disease: failure to thrive, irritability, vomiting and diarrhoea. A clinical diagnosis was made, without a duodenal biopsy. The symptoms responded well to a gluten-free diet, and she had then developed normally. She continued on a gluten-free diet until the age of nineteen, but then returned to a normal diet. At twenty, she underwent* *a normal pregnancy. It wasn't until a year later that she started to develop mild abdominal symptoms.*

A duodenal biopsy at this time indicated coeliac disease. This confirmed the childhood diagnosis which, theoretically, could have also been a gastro-intestinal infection or other food intolerance, that had improved fortuitously with the gluten-free diet. On returning to this diet, Tina's symptoms quickly improved.

Investigations
- **Blood Tests** These may reveal iron, folate or vitamin B12 deficiency.
- **Examination of faeces** As fat is poorly absorbed, the amount in the stools is greatly increased. Samples are taken over a period of five days as there is a wide daily variation in fat excretion. As this is an unpopular test with both patient and laboratory staff, it has largely been replaced by a small bowel biopsy.
- **Biopsy of the small intestine** This is a simple test carried out in all cases of suspected coeliac disease. A small metal capsule is passed into the duodenum, in conjunction with a narrow tube (fibreoptic endoscope). This enables rapid positioning of the capsule in the small intestine. A trigger is released, enabling a tiny blade in the capsule to slice off a minute piece of the lining of the small intestine. The whole procedure takes about ten minutes. If coeliac disease is present, examination under the microscope will reveal the characteristic smooth lining of the intestine. The millions of villi, instead of projecting out like fingers into the cavity of the ileum, are in fact totally flat.

Management of coeliac disease
In principle, the management of coeliac disease is simple: all gluten must be excluded from the diet. In practice, however, this is complicated by the fact that gluten is present in so many foodstuffs. The smallest amounts can cause the symptoms to recur. While wheat and rye products obviously contain gluten, it may also be hidden in many sauces, gravies and stock cubes.

Problems associated with the gluten-free diet
Whilst omitting gluten from the diet brings total relief of the symptoms of coeliac disease and the restoration of the lining of the intestine, it is not always an easy diet to follow. Quite apart from inadvertently eating

gluten, other problems may arise, such as weight loss or gain and constipation. I provide a counselling session after three months to check the progress of a patient who suffers from this condition.

Julie, a seventeen year old school girl, had been diagnosed with coeliac disease at the beginning of her A level year. After a month on the diet, she looked much healthier but was concerned about putting on too much weight. This had occurred because of improved absorption as a result of the renewal of the villi in the lining of the small intestine. She had also become constipated as she had stopped eating cereals containing bran, because of their gluten content. I suggested defatted rice bran, or soya bran as suitable alternatives.

Some patients may develop a fear of eating, due to the restrictions of the diet and may actually lose weight. In such cases, I encourage a diet consisting of fresh meat, vegetables, fish and fruit to which other safe foods can gradually be added.

The implications of a gluten-free diet are particularly serious for teenage patients. Julie was understandably resentful of the restrictions it imposed on her. Teenagers and young adults often remain clinically well when they stray from their diet, which can tempt them to abandon the diet. Eventually, problems such as diarrhoea and anaemia will creep up on them, particularly during times of stress. In Julie's case, the trigger was the increased pressure of her approaching A levels.

Communicating effectively with people who are in their teens can be tricky. For this reason, I refer all teenagers diagnosed with coeliac disease both to the counsellor and the dietitian in our practice. Since I have adopted this policy, I have noticed a remarkable difference in the attitude of such patients and their compliance to the diet. This was in fact the case with Julie who remained positive and cheerful throughout the initial stages of the management of the disorder.

Hopefully a cure for coeliac disease will eventually be found, which will remove the need for the special diet. While the clinical features, pathological appearances and treatment of the condition are well understood, the precise reason for being sensitive to gluten remains elusive. Some significant facts, however, have been established. It appears the disease may be due to a deficiency in the body's immune system, rendering it unable to cope with a certain molecule present in gluten. This molecule is then treated as a harmful substance by the immune system (the body's natural defence), which then tries to eliminate it from the body. It is expected that in the next few years, a greater understanding of the processes of the immune system will be achieved, furthering the development of a cure.

The Coeliac Society offers invaluable help to the sufferer, giving advice on how to live a happy life without gluten, which foods to avoid and a list of gluten-free products. It is important to remember that many of these are available on prescription, including gluten-free biscuits, flour, bread and pasta. Their address is listed at the back of the book, in the useful addresses section (page 213).

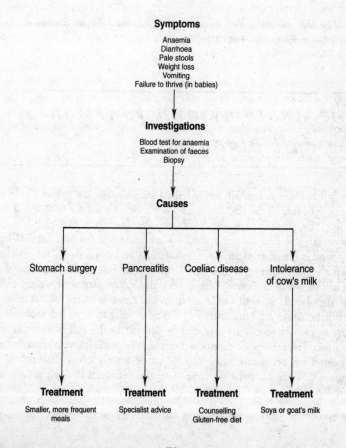

TREATMENT PLAN FOR MALABSORPTION

Symptoms

Anaemia
Diarrhoea
Pale stools
Weight loss
Vomiting
Failure to thrive (in babies)

↓

Investigations

Blood test for anaemia
Examination of faeces
Biopsy

↓

Causes

Stomach surgery	Pancreatitis	Coeliac disease	Intolerance of cow's milk
Treatment	**Treatment**	**Treatment**	**Treatment**
Smaller, more frequent meals	Specialist advice	Counselling Gluten-free diet	Soya or goat's milk

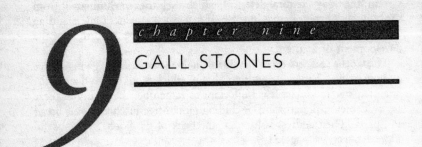

chapter nine

GALL STONES

❛ I've this terrible pain, doctor, just below my ribs, as if someone is twisting a knife into me. ❜

The anatomy and function of the gall bladder

The gall bladder is a small, pear-shaped sac situated just under the liver, on the right side of the abdomen, and is responsible for concentrating and storing bile. Bile is actually made in the liver but the gall bladder concentrates it five to ten times, by absorbing water and salt. When fatty food is eaten, the gall bladder contracts and its contents are expelled down the bile duct into the duodenum. The bile then emulsifies fat, helping to break it down. Bile is very thick, consisting of water, salts, cholesterol and pigment made up from the remains of red blood cells. If the bile becomes too concentrated, it may solidify to form gall stones – as many as twenty to twenty five can be present in the gall bladder at any one time. The stones are composed of the three main constituents in bile (although on occasions, they can be made purely of cholesterol or of pigment). What happens to these stones, determines the symptoms felt by the patient.

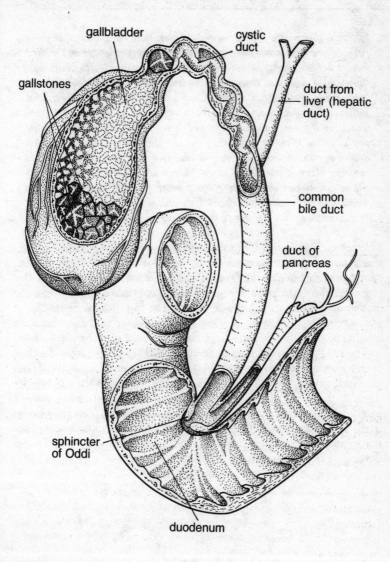

Figure 9.1   The gall bladder showing gall stones

Acute symptoms

Judith, a thirty nine year old mother of four, rang me one night in great pain. When I examined her a little later, she was very tender on the right side of her abdomen, just under the ribs. She explained the pain had started as a dull ache three hours previously but had suddenly become very severe, making her vomit. There was no doubt that Judith was suffering from gall stones and the first thing to do was to relieve her pain. Vomiting is a common feature of gall stones, so it was impossible in the initial period to give her tablets by mouth. I therefore injected her with a dose of morphine, which not only removed the pain, but also allowed her to sleep. When I returned to Judith's home later that morning, she was sitting up in bed and looking much more like her normal self. The vomiting had stopped and, although she still had an ache under her ribs, it was nothing like the agony she had experienced during the night.

In cases such as Judith's, the suddenness and severity of pain indicates that a stone has become stuck in the neck (or exit) of the gall bladder, completely obstructing the flow of bile. In an attempt to overcome this blockage, the muscles of the gall bladder contracted fiercely, causing intense and constant pain (biliary colic). The injection of morphine, as well as relieving the agony and allowing the patient to rest, also relaxes the muscles so the offending gall stone can drop back into the gall bladder.

The pain is often referred to the back and tip of the right shoulder blade. Vomiting occurs in most cases, rendering initial treatment of pain more difficult. If the gall stone does not drop back into the gall bladder quickly, the build up of bile can spill into the bloodstream, causing jaundice (which typically causes a yellow skin colouring. The gall bladder swells as the pressure of the bile increases, and after about twenty four hours, infection usually develops. The patient becomes very ill and develops a high temperature.

Chronic symptoms

Brenda, who is forty five, works in a local cake shop, just down the road from our surgery. Brenda had experienced intermittent episodes of pain and discomfort on the right side of her abdomen and persistent nausea after eating. She had developed a liking for cream cakes, which were a perk of her job, but in the past few months these had increasingly produced aches in her stomach. She finally came to the surgery when she began vomiting, her urine had become very dark, and her stools, much lighter. Wind had started to be an embarrassing problem, especially during the day at work.

On examination, the upper right side of Brenda's abdomen was very tender, although the rest of it felt normal. There was a yellowish tinge to her skin and the conjunctivae (the whites of the eyes) were distinctly jaundiced. The only other feature of note was that Brenda was about three stone overweight.

I explained to her that she was suffering from a common presentation of gall stones where the gall bladder becomes inflamed leading to pain, vomiting, jaundice, and a persistent intolerance of fatty food. These are similar symptoms to those of the acute form, but nothing like as severe.

Gall stones occur in about ten per cent of the population and are four times more common in women than in men. Classically, they arise in fair, fertile, middle-aged women, who have a tendency to be overweight. A high-fat diet increases the amount and concentration of bile which encourages the formation of gall stones and can increase the pressure in the gall bladder. It has been noted that fair people form much less bile, than those who have dark skin (gall bladder disease is very rare, for example, in Africa). This may simply be explained by a healthier diet (containing plenty of fruit and far less fat), compared to that in the West, and may in fact have little to do with skin colouring.

Harry, a fifty two year old man, experienced similar discomfort, with the pain also radiating to the right shoulder blade. This occurs because the sensory nerves to the gall bladder and the shoulder originate from the same area in the spinal cord. One morning, after a restless night, Harry noticed his skin looked yellow, so he came to the surgery as soon as we opened. One glance showed that he was quite jaundiced.

In cases such as these, a gall stone becomes stuck, not in the neck of the gall bladder (as in Judith's case), but in the bile duct (the tube carrying the bile downwards into the duodenum). The bile (which is yellow in colour) collects behind the stone, until it eventually reaches the level where it spills over into the bloodstream, causing the characteristic yellow colouring. If the flow of bile becomes blocked, then the digestion and absorption of fat is reduced in the gut, giving stools a pale colour. Exactly the opposite happens to urine, where the excess of bile in the bloodstream is filtered through the kidneys, making the urine much darker than usual.

Investigations

Anyone suspected of having gall bladder problems should have an ultrasound scan of their abdomen. This reveals the whole biliary system clearly outlining any gall stones present. The scan can be carried out as an emergency, in acute cases. If jaundice is present, then the level of bilirubin (responsible for the yellow pigment in bile) can be measured with a simple blood test.

Conventional treatment

The only permanent, conventional treatment for troublesome gall stones, is an operation to remove the gall bladder, and any stones present in the bile duct (cholecystectomy). Recovery is rapid, but it still necessitates a week in hospital and six weeks off work. We can function perfectly normally without a gall bladder as bile is still produced by the liver, and passes straight down the bile duct into the duodenum.

A less intrusive procedure is a laparoscopic cholecystectomy, where the operation is performed using a flexible endoscope, which has a light, a snare and some scissors. A small incision about ½ inch long is made and the tube passed through it. The endoscope permits the whole procedure to be viewed on a video screen. The gall bladder is then carefully freed from its structures and removed. Only one stitch is required and it is often possible to go home the following day. This type of operation is becoming more common but, as it is relatively new, not all surgeons have extensive experience in this technique.

Attempts are currently being made to perfect a laser treatment, where the stones are destroyed without damage to the surrounding tissues, but so far this has been largely ineffective.

It is important to remember that operations should not be undertaken simply for the presence of gall stones, because, in many people, they never give trouble. Surgery should be reserved for patients who have suffered one, or more, attacks of acute pain, or who have a long history of nausea, intolerance of fatty foods and continuous aching. Jaundice is, in itself, not a sufficient reason to operate as gall stones can often pass into the gut spontaneously. The build up of bile (which is responsible for this condition) therefore clears itself.

Non-surgical treatment involves the management of acute attacks and any infection that may develop. If a stone becomes lodged in the neck of the gall bladder, then initially a painkiller of morphine's strength is usually needed. An antispasmodic injection is given at the same time to ease the colic, which is combined with an antiemetic to quell the vomiting. Antibiotics should be used whenever fever is present. These are usually first injected and taken thereafter by mouth, if the sickness has settled.

However, there are times when an operation is unavoidable. Sometimes a stone stuck in the gall bladder neck will not fall back into the gall bladder, or a stone in the bile duct becomes firmly jammed. In situations such as these, immediate treatment should be given to prevent serious complications, such as infection or perforation. Surgical removal may be the only way of permanently resolving the problem. In others, the gall bladder may thicken through years of irritation by the stones, and here, surgical removal instantly improves the quality of life of the sufferer.

These conditions, however, are uncommon. Cholecystectomies are carried out in their thousands every week, but I suspect that they may not all be vitally necessary. That is not to say I would not advise an operation where it is absolutely necessary but I am one of an increasing number of doctors who prefer to try non-invasive treatments wherever possible, before resorting to the surgeon's knife.

Alternative therapies

DIET

The cornerstone of management is a low-fat diet, which reduces the need for the gall bladder to expel bile into the intestine. This type of diet is, in any case, a healthy one which can benefit anyone, regardless of the presence of gall stones. When the pain becomes severe, all dairy products and animal fats should be excluded, while cereals and raw vegetables should be eaten in large quantities. Fish and chicken can usually be tolerated (with the skin removed) but should be cooked without using animal fats.

As the effect of fats on the gall bladder varies from person to person, it may be possible to reintroduce some food which contains fat, once the symptoms have disappeared. Eggs are a classic example, as they can be tolerated by about half of all gall stone sufferers. Since biliary stasis (stagnation of the bile) is believed to favour stone formation, a moderate intake of uncooked fat is permitted (such as milk, butter and cream cheese) as these will promote the drainage of the gall bladder and its ducts.

CALORIE-CONTROLLED DIET

Many people who suffer from gall stones are considerably above their recommended weight. In such cases, a calorie-controlled diet is essential. A low-fat diet will help to maintain weight at a satisfactory level.

EXERCISE

A sluggish lifestyle leads to the sluggish functioning of the body, including a slower flow of bile. Regular exercise each day, even if it is only a twenty minute walk, will help tone the gall bladder muscles.

ACUPUNCTURE

Where the pain is particularly severe, I will often use acupuncture as a treatment. The aim of acupuncture is to restore the energy flow or *Chi* in the affected channels (see Chapter 3). In gall bladder pain, an obstruction in the gall bladder and liver channels occurs which may overlap into the

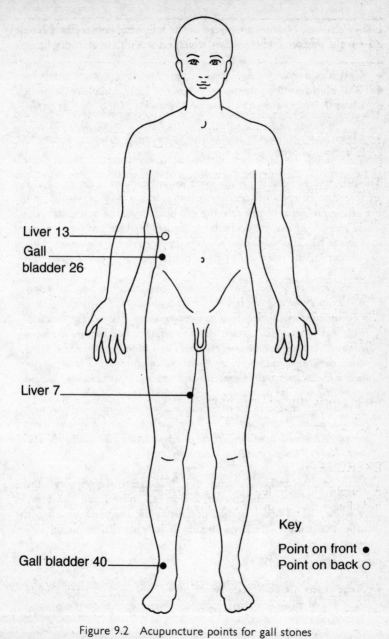

Figure 9.2 Acupuncture points for gall stones

kidney channel. Needles are placed at the following points (the Chinese express the measurements in *Cun*, which is the width of an index finger):

- **Gall bladder 26** 6 cun lateral to the navel on the right side;
- **Gall bladder 40** on the outer side of the foot just below the ankle;
- **Liver 7** 2 cun below the knee on the inside of the leg just behind the tibia;
- **Liver 13** on the outer side of the abdomen, 1 cun below the lowermost border of the rib cage.

The principle of needling is the same for any condition, in that needles are placed at the appropriate acupuncture points as close as possible to the site of the problem, in this case the gall bladder and also at distal points where the *Chi* enters the body. Both the gall bladder and liver channels start in the legs and work their way up the front of the abdomen. This is the reason for the selection of these points (see Figure 9.2, page 87).

Harry came to see me with acute pain and jaundice, two symptoms which can be successfully treated with acupuncture. Four needles were gently inserted and stimulated for twenty minutes. The relief of pain was rapid but it recurred, though not as severely, when the needles were removed. As each acupuncture channel has a branch to the ear, I left a small, metal stud in the ear (see Figure 3.2 on page 15). The use of ear studs is a vital part of the therapist's armoury and is particularly effective in conditions where pain is of an intermittent nature. Harry was able to stimulate this stud with his index finger whenever he felt the start of a painful spasm. Harry settled well and only required four treatment sessions to settle his pain completely. As acupuncture also relaxes the bile duct, Harry's stone passed spontaneously.

The sudden onset and severe nature of gall bladder pain often prevents the use of homoeopathic remedies, which are a little slow to act. However, in cases where the pain is bearable, homoeopathic remedies are often the treatment of choice. Effective remedies in an acute situation are:

HOMOEOPATHY

- **Argentum nit 6c** is suitable for persistent, nagging pain. People who are of an anxious and volatile nature experience the best results with this treatment;

- **Belladonna 6c** is a good alternative where the person is normally lively and cheerful;
- **Berberis 30c** can be used where there is a tearing pain right around the abdomen (which is made worse by movement), where there is jaundice, nausea and vomiting. It is most suited to people with a confident personality;
- **China 30c** is recommended where pain is lessened by bending double, where the sufferer prefers to move around (rather than sit still), and where there is much flatulence (which does not relieve the pain). It suits those of a nervous disposition.

Any homoeopathic remedy has the great advantage that it can be taken when vomiting is present, as the tablets dissolve under the tongue. I usually recommend them to be taken every hour for the first few doses, cutting back to four times a day, when the symptoms start to settle.

At the time of her greatest agony, Judith would not have worried whatever treatment I had given her. The dose of morphine was a very welcome relief. However, the following morning, she asked me if there was any natural treatment she could take by mouth. As Judith was of an outgoing, jolly personality, Berberis was the choice for her.

On the other hand, Brenda's gall bladder problem was long standing, with low-grade and constant pain. She described herself as a worrier, impulsive, quickly irritated and generally pessimistic. These features of her personality, together with her chronic pain, made her suitable for Argentum nit (taken three times daily).

HERBAL TREATMENT

- **Berberis** There is considerable overlap between homoeopathy and herbal medicine in the management of an inflamed gall bladder, as berberis is often used in both specialities. The herb, berberis, stimulates bile flow and eases liver congestion. 15 gm of the herb (either the bark or the root), is added to 600 mls of water and heated to near-boiling point for fifteen minutes. The mixture is drained and drunk by the cupful, three times a day. Alternatively 8 mls of the tincture can be taken each day.
- **Fringe tree** The herb, fringe tree, is also effective but it can be difficult to obtain. It is taken in the same way as berberis.

- **Peppermint** This is much easier to buy than fringe tree. Although not specific to the gall bladder, it is soothing to the stomach and most valuable in any situation where there is pain and vomiting. Peppermint can either be made into a fresh infusion (see Chapter 13) or is available in tea bag form from all health food stores.

Both conventional and alternative medicine have a great deal to offer in the treatment of gall stones and their accompanying problems and are best used in combination.

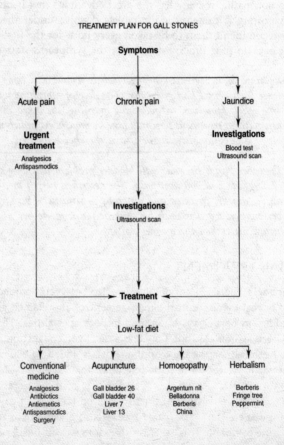

TREATMENT PLAN FOR GALL STONES

Symptoms

Acute pain   Chronic pain   Jaundice

Urgent treatment

Analgesics
Antispasmodics

Investigations

Blood test
Ultrasound scan

Investigations

Ultrasound scan

Treatment

Low-fat diet

Conventional medicine	Acupuncture	Homoeopathy	Herbalism
Analgesics	Gall bladder 26	Argentum nit	Berberis
Antibiotics	Gall bladder 40	Belladonna	Fringe tree
Antiemetics	Liver 7	Berberis	Peppermint
Antispasmodics	Liver 13	China	
Surgery			

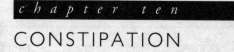

chapter ten

CONSTIPATION

' My mother always said you won't stay healthy if you don't open your bowels every day. '

There is more unnecessary worry about constipation, than virtually any other medical problem. For some unknown reason, people in the West have become obsessed with their bowel habits, ending up addicted to drugs that open them. I find myself reassuring patients that they do not need to be taking continual doses of laxatives, almost every day. There is a wide variation in the frequency of defaecation. Ninety per cent of people in Britain, for example, open their bowels between twice a day and five times a week. A minority, do so on fewer occasions. These people accept their habit as normal while, in contrast, a great many consider themselves constipated because they do not go every day. This misconception often stems from childhood and the rigid attitude of parents towards toilet training. A definition of constipation should not be centred on the infrequency of bowel movements. A better description would be: the production of hard stool which requires excessive straining to pass. The usual pattern of an individual's bowel movements may also be upset. This, in itself, is not an indication of constipation, however. Constipation occurs where the slow passage of stools through the large intestine, results in greater amounts of water being absorbed, making them dry and hard.

Causes

- **Diet** Approximately ninety five per cent of all cases of constipation in the West are caused by lack of fibre in the diet, which is often associated with insufficient fluid intake. Fibre (plant substances which are not digested) is very important for the proper working of the intestines. It passes unchanged through the intestine where it absorbs water, increases the bulk of undigested food, and improves the functioning of the muscles of the large intestine, preventing constipation and straining. In the West, diets are low in fibre because food has often been processed in a way which removes and destroys fibre, for example white flour, where the fibre rich outer layers have been removed in the milling process. In addition, there is a tendency to eat insufficient fruit and vegetables.
- **Drugs** Certain medicines have side-effects which cause constipation. These commonly include antidepressants, painkillers and iron tablets.
- **Pregnancy** The hormone changes of pregnancy reduce the effectiveness of bowel muscle contraction, slowing the passage of faeces along the intestines.
- **The menopause** Again, hormone changes may also affect the muscles of the large intestine, resulting in constipation.
- **Age** With advancing age, the muscles of the intestine become weaker and take longer to push the faeces through the bowel.
- **Ignoring the urge to defaecate** Many patients who suffered from constipation have repeatedly ignored the urge to defaecate when their rectum was full. This eventually reduces their sensitivity to the defaecating reflex. In the majority of patients, the reasons for denying this urge are sociological rather than medical, such as embarrassment in requesting to leave classrooms or places of work, or a dislike of public lavatories. Painful anal conditions such as piles or fissures may force sufferers to open their bowels as infrequently as possible.
- **Lack of exercise** Very few people who exercise regularly have constipation, as long as they replace the fluid lost during the exertion. A sedentary lifestyle reduces the tone in the intestinal muscles. It is commonly seen in old people in nursing homes who are immobile.

- **Psychological** Anxiety, stress and tension can often contribute to the condition.
- **Thyroid disease** The thyroid gland determines the rate at which the body functions. An underactive gland will slow the muscle contractions in the large intestine, resulting in constipation. Other symptoms of this condition include: excess weight gain, thickening of the skin, hair loss and extreme tiredness.
- **Bowel cancer** Although this is the most serious cause of constipation, it is thankfully the least common. A tumour growing into the cavity of the bowel will partially block the passage of faeces, causing constipation. Any sudden onset of constipation for no apparent reason, especially if it is accompanied by significant weight loss, will need investigating to exclude cancer. Early diagnosis of a tumour is vital, so that curative treatment can be given immediately.

Investigations

Most people do not require any investigations as the cause of the constipation is obvious. However, in cases where the onset of constipation is sudden and accompanied by significant weight loss, investigations are essential.

SIMPLE EXAMINATION

Normally, when feeling the abdomen, it is not possible to feel the large intestine. In constipation, however, the whole length of the bowel is often distended as it is full of hard faeces. If there is no sign of any other swellings or lumps, bowel cancer is unlikely.

RECTAL EXAMINATION

This involves the gentle placing of a finger into the anus and rectum. Though many people find this procedure embarrassing, it is necessary because it reveals the consistency of the faeces. The rectum is usually empty but, if a person is constipated, it is full. The faeces are hard and may either be large in volume or small and hard, like stones. Piles around

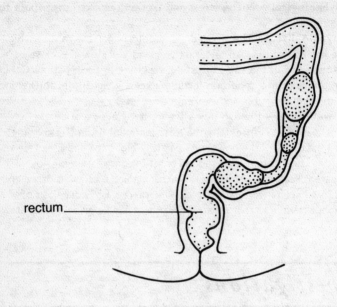

rectum

Figure 10.1   Constipation

the anus or a rectal tumour which is hard or ulcerated, can also be discovered in this way.

BARIUM ENEMA

Where constipation is obvious, but no cause can actually be found, a barium enema is essential. A small amount of barium sulphate is inserted into the rectum via a narrow tube. This compound is radio-opaque and shows up white on the X-ray. It outlines the whole of the large bowel up to where it starts at the caecum. Any tumours can be identified either as an irregular outline, or as a narrowing in the bowel causing partial obstruction to the flow of barium.

COLONOSCOPY

If the X-rays indicate any of the above conditions, then a colonoscopy is necessary. A small flexible tube is passed through the anus and up the large intestine. The distal end of this tube has a light fitted to it whilst the proximal end has an eyepiece. By looking through this the examiner can view the lining of the bowel directly. Any tumours will be clearly visible.

Sid, a seventy five year old man, experienced a sudden onset of constipation. There seemed to be no reason for this as he had always had regular, bowel movements every day. His stools had become hard in the past two months, and he had noticed he was losing weight. He had also not changed his lifestyle in any way. It was therefore essential to exclude a bowel cancer. I referred Sid to a specialist at the hospital for investigations.

Happily for Sid, all his tests were completely normal, so it was certain a cancer was not lurking in his intestines. I concluded his constipation was from a number of factors, including lack of fibre in his diet, immobility, too little exercise, insufficient fluid intake and a general reluctance to open his bowels as the passage of hard stools was uncomfortable. The weight loss was likely to have been from a decreased appetite which he had not mentioned previously. The surprising thing was that Sid's constipation had come on so suddenly, but this can happen – at times our bowels seem to have a mind of their own, and do not always behave exactly as expected!

Management

LIFESTYLE CHANGES

Simple changes often produce the best results. Often all that is needed is to be aware of the factors which exacerbate constipation. Regular daily exercise should be taken (this need only be a brisk walk for half an hour or, if more vigorous exercise is preferred, squash or cycling are effective. Long periods of immobility must be avoided. It is also most important to respond appropriately to the defaecation urge.

DIET

In most people, normal bowel movement can be restored by switching to high-fibre foods. It is often unnecessary to take bulking laxatives.

Wholegrains like wholemeal bread, fresh fruit and raw vegetables are particularly recommended. It is far better to eat food in its natural state rather than just sprinkle bran on top of a refined carbohydrate. However, bran can be helpful as an interim measure. Other foods with natural laxative properties can be added, such as dried fruit like prunes and apricots. Fortunately high-fibre diets are becoming more popular and there are the many books on the market which provide a wide variety of recipes.

Debbie is a twenty five year old computer operator who had seen me three months previously with chronic constipation. I had recommended a high-fibre diet but she returned with little improvement, certain there was something seriously wrong with her. She was unconvinced by my reassurance so I arranged a barium enema, which did not reveal any abnormalities. Debbie then bought herself a high-fibre cookery book which listed easy-to-make, high-fibre dishes. Debbie's fibre consumption increased even more and her constipation was relieved.

People's intestines are as different from one another as their outward appearance: what may be a high-fibre diet for one colon, can be too much for a second and too little for a third to cope with. We all need a diet which is sufficiently rich in fibre to avoid constipation. On average 20–30 gm of fibre is sufficient but this of course varies from individual to individual. If switching to wholefoods is not sufficient, then bran can be added to the diet, although it is important to start slowly, usually with one to two teaspoons per day. The dose can be gradually increased. Large quantities of bran suddenly appearing in the bowel can cause the bacteria living there to form quantities of gas which distend the abdomen, leading to bloating and anti-social flatulence.

Joan came to the surgery on a very busy Monday morning, suffering from constipation. I must have convinced her of the need for a high-fibre diet, because she took her husband straight to the nearest health food shop and purchased a generous supply of high-fibre foods. They went home and began to eat them enthusiastically. They were both so embarrassed by the wind they produced that it took them nearly a year to come back to see me!

It is for this reason that fibre should be gradually added to the diet, continuing slowly until the desired effect is produced. A fuller description of a high-fibre diet is included in the section on Diverticulitis (page 155).

The diet should be supplemented with vitamin B1 (10 mg daily) and magnesium aspartate (1.5 gm daily) as these help to stimulate the intestinal muscles.

FLUID INTAKE

An increased fluid intake is almost as important as a high-fibre diet. Most constipated people drink far too little – intake should be at least three pints daily. Alcohol should not be included in this measurement as it dehydrates the body. In fact, alcoholics often suffer from severe constipation.

Conventional treatment

BULKING AGENTS

Most patients begin to eat sufficient amounts of fibre when they are constipated but some do not realise this should be for every day of their lives. Some even refuse, or are unable to cope with, the diet. It is in these cases that a proprietary bulking agent can be used. There are a large number on the market made mostly from ispaghula, sterculia or methylcellulose. The appropriate dose is that which brings the desired result. Again, these bulking agents are not usually an intermittent treatment, but are mainly used long-term.

LAXATIVES

A professor who taught me at medical college used to say it was never necessary to give a laxative except for patients who were seriously ill and taking morphine. This drug causes severe constipation. My experience as a general practitioner, has proved him to be wrong, however. Some patients are not relieved by fibre or fibre supplements. This is most likely to be because of poor muscular action (i.e. a lazy bowel). Laxative therapy can help to improve this condition. There are three groups:

- **Stimulant laxatives** These stimulate the intestine to contract and expel the stool. They are best used occasionally as they can damage the supply of nerves in the intestines. Drugs in this category include bisacodyl and senna.

- **Osmotic laxatives** These soften and expand the stool by keeping waste water in the intestine. This stimulates the intestine to contract and the stool is passed. The most commonly used is lactulose. Although different laxatives suit different people, I usually recommend this drug as it is effective and has the fewest side-effects. The usual dose is two teaspoons twice daily (although double this amount can be taken if required).

- **Stool softeners** This type of laxative softens the stool and impede water absorption in the large intestine. Examples are docusate or liquid paraffin.

Inappropriate use of laxatives

Abuse of laxatives is common and, must be avoided at all costs. Many patients become convinced they have an unsatisfactory bowel habit and, as a consequence, go to the local chemist or supermarket and buy laxatives. This is without paying any attention to their diet or fibre intake.

Bridget was one such person. She was a forty six year old woman who had become constipated at the onset of the menopause. By the time she came to see me, she had been taking laxatives for over a year. She believed that she would not open her bowels for several weeks if she stopped taking them. She wrongly attributed a multitude of symptoms (such as headaches and lethargy) to her sluggish bowel function. Bridget had probably been ill-advised during childhood, leading to her routine usage of laxatives. However, a good number of these contain powerful drugs and are not to be played around with. She had been taking senna (which can damage the nerve supply to the bowel if used for a long period of time).

Bridget's bowel needed re-educating. I replaced the senna she had been taking with lactulose (which holds water in the intestine) for a few days. Bridget then increased her dietary fibre and took a spoonful of Fybogel (Ispaghula) each day. I warned her it would take several weeks, perhaps months for her bowel to resume its normal, regular function. Bridget persevered very well and has now fully recovered.

The routine usage of laxatives can provoke a condition called cathartic colon, where the intestines, driven for several years by stimulant purgatives, finally fail to respond and the bowels refuse to open at all. Enemas are often needed to clear the blocked colon. Stimulant laxatives (such as senna) may also empty the bowel completely and it can then take several days for it to fill again. Anyone who is obsessed with a daily bowel movement, will assume they are still constipated and take further doses of laxative. Stimulating an empty bowel can cause severe cramping pains.

It is nevertheless important to remember that elderly people, who have taken laxatives sometimes for twenty to thirty years, have less of a chance of successfully converting to a new regime. In such cases, it may be necessary to continue with the stimulant laxative, combined with intermittent enemas or suppositories.

Alternative therapies

As with orthodox medicine, natural therapy is based largely upon lifestyle changes and increased fibre in the diet. In addition to these changes, all the major complimentary specialities can be successfully used, instead of taking potentially harmful commercial laxatives.

HOMOEOPATHY

In homoeopathy, constipation is regarded as a constitutional problem. The choice of remedy therefore depends upon personality, as well as the disorder. There are a bewildering number of remedies on the market, but, however, the following are suitable for a wide range of personalities:

- **Alumina;**
- **Nux vomica;**
- **Plumbum;**
- **Sulphur.**

These should all be taken in the potency of 6c, although this is not vital if the shop only has 30c in stock.

Grace was sixty three when she first came to see me, with an eighteen month history of increasing constipation. She had a continual urge to pass stools but usually nothing came, or they were not completely eliminated. Grace had tried various laxatives over the previous year and was now taking steadily increasing doses of senna. She is a tall, thin dark lady who described herself as inclined to be impatient and easily irritated. Her symptoms were worse at night and improved with warmth. The treatment of choice for her was Nux vomica in 6c. She was slowly able to replace senna with this remedy.

Neil, who is twenty three, came to see me with severe rectal pain associated with hard stools which were passed every two to three days. On examination he had a crack in the anal wall from straining (anal fissure. There were also a few small piles present. His stools were dark, large, dry and hard. He occasionally noticed a small amount of diarrhoea, leaking from his anus. Neil described himself as a deep-thinking, rather nervous individual. Sulphur in the 6c potency, combined with extra fluid intake helped soften his stools. This remedy is also particularly suited to children.

Doreen, at the age of seventy, considered herself incurable as she had suffered with constipation for many years and had already tried a homoeopathic remedy from the local health food shop which had not helped her condition, but it was obviously not the correct one. Doreen suffered with sharp griping pains and straining, only producing small hard, black, stone-like stools. Doreen described herself as self-confident, very outgoing and sociable. She mixed easily with people and enjoyed laughing. I prescribed Plumbum 6c which certainly helped.

Duncan described his stools as soft and clay-like, which were sometimes covered in mucus. He had no desire to open his bowels until his rectum was completely full and had the feeling that stools were getting caught up, on the left side of the abdomen. Duncan described himself as a quiet type who liked reading and listening to the radio. He preferred the arts to sport and exercise. A prescription for Alumina 6c improved his bowel function.

As always, when seeking a homoeopathic remedy, it is important to seek the advice of a qualified practitioner, as it is often difficult to select the correct one for your personality and symptoms.

HERBAL TREATMENT

Excellent natural laxatives are available for the relief of constipation although, again, they will be largely ineffective without the diet and lifestyle changes.

Rhubarb

Perhaps the most effective remedy, it is certainly the easiest to obtain. It can be used in its natural form and as dry powder, which is available from most health food stores. It can also be taken as a tincture (2 mls, three times daily). Rhubarb contains anthraquinones which irritate the gut lining, causing it to move the stools along more rapidly. Unlike Senna, there is no risk of damage to the bowel's nerve supply. Rhubarb is best taken as an infusion. 10 to 15 gm of the herb to one pint of water, is steamed for twenty minutes, then strained. This can be drunk by the cupful, morning and night.

Linseed

This has been used as a bulking laxative since Greek times. Hippocrates recommended the seeds for inflammation of the bowel and constipation. In France, during the eighth century, Charlemagne passed laws requiring the consumption of these seeds to keep his subjects healthy and regular in habit. The seeds can be chewed or swallowed with water. The dose is one or two tablespoons with two glasses of water, each day. The seeds gently swell up in the bowel to produce a bulking laxative. They can be mixed with muesli, porridge, honey or soft cheese and eaten at breakfast. The seeds can be soaked overnight in water and then taken, however this is not as effective as swallowing them dry.

Guelder Rose

This is a smooth muscle relaxant which is most effective where constipation causes cramping pain. An alternative name for guelder rose is in fact cramp bark. It is taken as a tincture (2 mls, twice daily).

ACUPUNCTURE

Many people think of acupuncture only as a treatment of painful conditions, however it is used for many constitutional disorders, including constipation. Acupuncture is described fully in Chapter 3.

In Chinese medicine, the proper functioning of the bowel is considered dependent on the health of the small intestine from which it receives waste material. It also relies on an efficient stomach and spleen (the organs first called upon to extract the essence of the *Chi* energy from food. The treatment of constipation using acupuncture is not, therefore, confined to the needling of the bowel channel, but with the correction of all causative energy imbalances in the other channels including the small intestine, large intestine and stomach.

I only use acupuncture in the most resistant cases as a combination of dietary changes, homoeopathic medication and herbal remedies work so well and are more convenient. However, I sometimes teach acupressure (which the patient can carry out at home). Four points are used (see Figure 10.2). Each should be gently massaged for a few minutes at a time.

Management of specific conditions

FAECAL IMPACTION

Impaction of stools in the rectum is the result of severe constipation and is a common problem in the elderly. As many of us look after ageing relatives, it is a condition we need to know how to deal with.

> I was recently called out to one of the local nursing homes to see Hilda who was eighty three years old and had not moved her bowels for over a month. She had just left her own house and I therefore suspected it was the change of diet that had caused the problem. Examination of her abdomen revealed an easily palpable large intestine, with huge masses of faeces along its whole length. Some nursing homes are very helpful when it comes to the use of natural therapies and I was able to prescribe a combination of the homoeopathic remedy Plumbum, combined with some linseed seeds to be sprinkled on her food. One of the nursing staff gave her regular olive oil enemas to empty the bowel gradually. Fortunately Hilda's bowels slowly cleared without the need for orthodox laxatives.

If these measures are insufficient then a stimulant laxative such as senna is used and occasionally if all else fails it is necessary to remove the faeces digitally through the rectum.

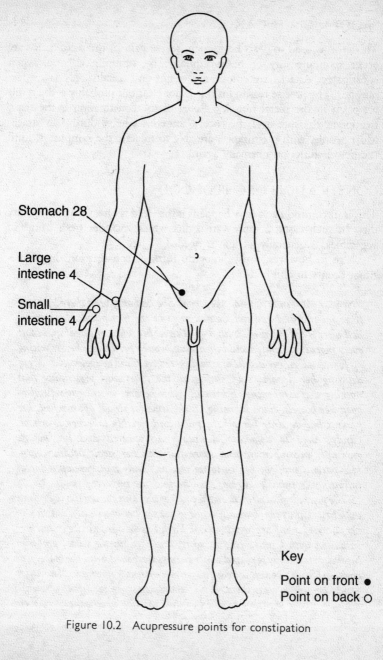

Figure 10.2 Acupressure points for constipation

PROCTALGIA FUGAX

This term is used to describe sudden, severe pain in the rectum. It may occur spontaneously or be precipitated by straining at stool when constipated. Attacks are common at night and usually only last a few minutes. The precise reason for this is not clear but probably is the result of spasm in the rectal muscles. Relief of the constipation is the main treatment. Pressure over the coccyx sometimes helps during an attack. Most people, with reassurance, are able to tolerate the symptoms, until the bowels function normally again.

CONSTIPATION IN CHILDHOOD

This is uncommon and only happens if the child is on a very poor quality diet. In such cases, a more varied diet which includes fresh fruit and vegetables, is generally all that is needed.

There is, however, a psychological form of constipation that sometimes occurs in children.

Five year old Cindy did not like school. She had only been there less than three months and had not wanted to go in the first place. Her parents had always fed her well, with a good sized breakfast of cereal and toast every morning. Cindy would then usually open her bowels before setting off for school. As her dislike of school increased, Cindy developed a way of delaying her departure by sitting on the toilet and pretending that nothing was happening. Eventually, this became a straight refusal to open her bowels. Each morning, as the time for school approached, her parents had to drag her off the toilet and forcibly take her to school. Cindy's urge to defaecate eventually disappeared and her bowels gradually became more and more full and her stools became hard. Her parents brought her in to see me, as Cindy had developed faecal incontinence from leakage of stool around the impacted stools.

The psychological element in the cause of the constipation has to be dealt with first. Cindy was basically refusing to open her bowels as a reaction to her parents forcing her to go to school. First, I asked our practice counsellor, in liaison with Cindy's teacher, to try and sort out the school problem. Second, gentle daily soap and water enemas were used until the bowel was clear, as Cindy's bowels were so full neither orthodox nor natural laxatives would be able to clear them. It was also necessary to modify the parents' attitude, in the way they handled Cindy's reaction to school and in their desire to keep their child's bowels regular.

It took a full three months of careful psychological handling before Cindy started to like going to school. It was only then that her bowel function returned to normal. I am pleased to say Cindy is now a happy child with plenty of friends at school.

While it is not a common problem, constipation in children must always be taken seriously as psychological factors usually play a significant role. Up to a few years ago, it was sometimes necessary to admit children with faecal impaction to hospital, both for enemas (to clear the bowel) and also in order to remove them (temporarily) from the possible underlying problems at home. Improved psychological services, such as practice counsellors, and a more sympathetic approach to parents' reactions, has meant that constipation in children can usually be managed in the home environment.

TREATMENT PLAN FOR CONSTIPATION

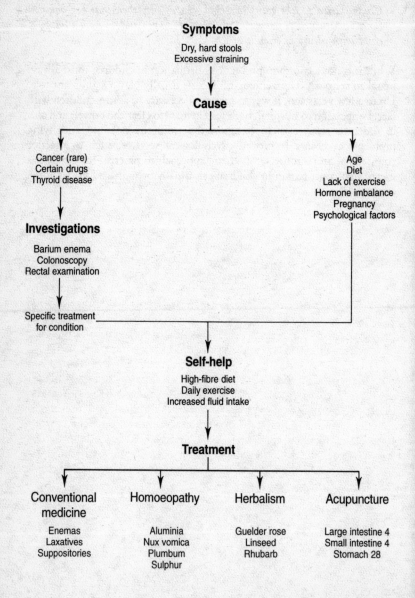

Symptoms

Dry, hard stools
Excessive straining

↓

Cause

Cancer (rare)
Certain drugs
Thyroid disease

Age
Diet
Lack of exercise
Hormone imbalance
Pregnancy
Psychological factors

↓

Investigations

Barium enema
Colonoscopy
Rectal examination

↓

Specific treatment
for condition

Self-help

High-fibre diet
Daily exercise
Increased fluid intake

↓

Treatment

Conventional medicine	Homoeopathy	Herbalism	Acupuncture
Enemas	Aluminia	Guelder rose	Large intestine 4
Laxatives	Nux vomica	Linseed	Small intestine 4
Suppositories	Plumbum	Rhubarb	Stomach 28
	Sulphur		

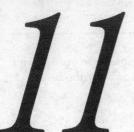

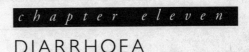

chapter eleven

DIARRHOEA

The major condition affecting the large intestine is acute diarrhoea, which can often be most unpleasant and debilitating. Diarrhoea can take many forms but the general definition is looseness of the stools, which may range in severity from semi-formed, to totally unformed, with a watery consistency. The looser the stool, the more distressing it is to the sufferer. There may, or may not, be increased frequency of bowel movement. Some people may believe they have diarrhoea when they simply have experienced an increase in frequency of a normally formed stool, perhaps accompanied by the passage of wind. This may be due to a slight increase in the muscle contractions in the large intestine, which may be related to a change in diet or anxiety. It may also be a warning of the onset of diarrhoea in the next few hours.

Under normal circumstances, undigested matter, as it enters the large intestine at the caecum, is in a fluid state. As it passes along towards the rectum, water is gradually reabsorbed. By the time stools are passed, they have become solid. Faeces are pushed along the large intestine by muscular contraction and if these contractions are too rapid, there is insufficient time for the water to be absorbed. A liquid stool is then passed (precisely the opposite occurs in constipation). Anything that makes the intestinal muscle become twitchy and overactive, will therefore produce diarrhoea.

Causes

For convenience diarrhoea can be subdivided into four main groups: acute, infective; traveller's; drug-related and chronic diarrhoea.

ACUTE, INFECTIVE DIARRHOEA

This undoubtedly is the most frequent cause of diarrhoea.

Numerous organisms can be responsible. Viral infections tend to affect groups of people – often causing epidemics in school children. The two most common are the rotavirus and the parvovirus. Although the symptoms are unpleasant, they are self-limiting and often clear spontaneously in twenty four to forty eight hours.

> *Keith is a thirty eight year old computer operator whom I visited at home one morning, when he was complaining of severe diarrhoea with the passage of watery motions every fifteen minutes. He also experienced nausea and vomiting, lassitude, headache, fever and shivering. He worked in a crowded office and said that several of his work colleagues were also suffering. This combination of factors all pointed to an infective cause.*

The main bacteria which produce diarrhoea are salmonella, shigella and campylobacter. Shigella is spread by contact with an infected stool or from faecal staining on clothes. The incubation period is two to four days. Diagnosis is confirmed by sending a stool sample to the pathology lab for culture. Although the person always looks terrible, admission to hospital is only necessary if severe dehydration occurs.

While shigella is caught by close contact with infected material, the bacteria salmonella infects food. The infection usually occurs in dairy products and meat (especially poultry) which is insufficiently cooked. Food from the deep freeze is particularly at risk if it hasn't properly thawed out. This type of infection is common in schools, restaurants and even hospitals. The incubation period is shorter than the other germs, usually between twelve and twenty four hours.

Symptoms are like those of shigella: copious diarrhoea containing blood and mucus. While the severest symptoms settle in two to three days, it may take several weeks before the bowel habit returns to normal.

Campylobacter is an organism which has emerged recently and is harboured by many animals including chickens, sheep, pigs, dogs and cats. Unpasteurised milk and untreated water have also been implicated in some outbreaks. Unlike other infections, there is an incubation period of three days before the diarrhoea starts, over which period symptoms including headache, muscle pains, a high temperature and shivering may occur. Diarrhoea lasts about forty eight hours and is watery with only occasional specks of blood. It is often accompanied by severe abdominal pain which may occasionally be mistaken for peritonitis. Colicky pain may persist for some weeks after the infection has cleared.

June, a nurse at our local hospital, woke with pains in her stomach in the middle of the night, which rapidly progressed to diarrhoea containing blood and mucus. Over the following few hours, the pain in her lower abdomen increased and she developed a constant desire to open the bowels (tenesmus). On examination June looked very poorly and had a low-grade temperature. Her abdomen was tender, mainly over the left side which is the part of the intestine usually affected by bacterial infections. As June is a nurse, constantly handling soiled clothes and bed linen, a shigella infection was most likely.

TRAVELLER'S DIARRHOEA

Thanks to the improvements which have been made in world travel, many more people travel abroad and this has led to the emergence of traveller's diarrhoea. Twenty per cent of travellers experience diarrhoea. In certain parts of the world (such as Egypt, Mexico and India), the incidence of this condition is much higher. Although most episodes are self-limiting, it can be a major inconvenience. No one wants to spend their holiday ill.

Jason went to Turkey with some friends to celebrate his eighteenth birthday. It was the first time he had been abroad. He spent the first two days lying in the hot sun on the beach, during the day, and drinking plenty of cold beers at the local discos, at night. However, three days into the holiday, he developed cramp-like abdominal pains and copious diarrhoea. He spent the next four days confined to his hotel room. Only on the last day did Jason feel any better and by then it was time to return home. The holiday had been a total disaster.

Many people have their holidays ruined by illness. The causative organism is nearly always a bug called E.Coli which produces a very nasty toxin. It is a bacteria that travellers have usually not been exposed to in the past and they are therefore particularly susceptible to it. This is particularly true of those who have not been abroad before.

Transmission is by the faecal-oral route, usually through the ingestion of contaminated food or drinking water, swimming pool water and, occasionally, seawater contaminated by sewage. Ice in drinks may also carry the bacteria.

My own practice has an advice sheet for all holidaymakers, however I suspect this is rarely followed, as most travellers find restrictive practices difficult to accept while they are supposed to be enjoying themselves. Business and professional travellers in particular, may find themselves unable to avoid eating with the local residents. You can't be too careful. In fact doctors are no more sensible in this than anyone else. Over half of the gastro-enterologists attending a recent conference in Mexico City developed traveller's diarrhoea – and they are supposed to be experts on the subject!

E.Coli is common in Mediterranean resorts but further afield (for example South America and India), there are a whole range of diarrhoea-producing organisms including viruses and parasites (such as Giardia). In a recent survey of travellers who passed through Katmandu after trekking in the Himalayas, over thirty five per cent of stools were found to be infected.

DRUG-RELATED DIARRHOEA

This is a well-recognised effect of some drug treatments. However, it is rarely severe except when it is a side-effect of certain antibiotics. The diarrhoea usually clears up when the drug is withdrawn. Occasionally, however, a condition called pseudomembranous colitis may occur. The most commonly implicated antibiotics are the Penicillin group, particularly Amoxycillin. The inflammatory condition is caused by the bacteria called clostridium difficile and is sometimes of such severity that hospital admission is required to correct the ensuing dehydration and chemical imbalance.

Where symptoms have coincided with starting a new medication, it is wise, if possible, to stop it and change to an alternative, even if you think the drug is probably not responsible. Common drugs causing mild diarrhoea are digoxin, indomethacin (Indocid) and mephanamic acid (Ponstan).

CHRONIC DIARRHOEA

Most cases of diarrhoea seen in the surgery are a result of one of the three causes given above. Occasionally, some patients develop chronic diarrhoea associated with some gastro-intestinal problem. This is much more gradual in onset and nowhere near as debilitating as acute diarrhoea. Most of these are dealt with in other chapters and include:

- **Irritable bowel syndrome** In these cases, diarrhoea is intermittent and associated with colicky pain and abdominal distension. (See Chapter 12);
- **Alcohol** Excessive intake over a long period leads to mild diarrhoea;
- **Crohn's disease and ulcerative colitis** These are serious conditions of the bowel and are covered in detail in Chapter 14;
- **Malabsorption** Certain foodstuffs are not absorbed into the bloodstream, creating abnormal stools which may be loose (see Chapter 8);
- **Surgery** In the past, operations for stomach ulcers would frequently upset the rest of the intestines. Although these operations are rare these days, there are still many people alive who had them carried out twenty or thirty years ago and still feel the effects;
- **Endocrine causes** An overactive thyroid gland can often be associated with diarrhoea. This usually settles as soon as the gland function returns to normal;
- **Tumours** Cancer of the colon can instigate diarrhoea. It is worth noting that very few cases of diarrhoea with bleeding are from a malignant tumour and tumours in the large intestine are rare causes of diarrhoea (see Chapter 16).

Diagnosis

If the doctor spends enough time with a patient, it is usually possible to determine the cause of the diarrhoea simply from the description of their symptoms. The examination and investigations are merely confirmatory.

People with diarrhoea should be asked the following questions:

- Have they travelled outside their own country in the preceding few months?

- Has their diet changed in the week before the illness, have they eaten out or had any unusual foods?
- Are other members of the family or close colleagues suffering as well?
- For patients who live or eat in a large institution – has there been a sudden occurrence of gastro-intestinal symptoms in any of their fellow residents?
- Has there been blood in the diarrhoea?
- Has there been severe abdominal pain?
- Did significant weight loss occur before the diarrhoea started?
- Has the patient vomited?
- Have any operations been carried out in the past?
- Are any drugs being taken?
- Is stress excessive at present?

Derek, a fifty seven year old solicitor, came to see me with a four week history of diarrhoea, accompanied by occasional vomiting and cramping abdominal pain. He had been to India on holiday and the diarrhoea had started about a week after his return. Derek had lost about a stone in weight. With his work he often ate business lunches and went to company dinners. He had recently begun to notice streaks of blood in the stools.

My initial thoughts pointed towards an infective cause from his holiday in India. However, it was important to consider the other possibilities. It could have been an infection from eating out in this country, although the four week history was rather long. In addition, Derek has suffered from an irregular heartbeat controlled with Digoxin, which is a drug known to cause diarrhoea. However, he had taken this for two years without any problem. The weight loss and streaking of blood could perhaps point to a more serious underlying cause, such as a tumour. While the vacation was still the most likely reason for the diarrhoea, it was necessary to carry out some tests to confirm this.

Investigations

STOOL SAMPLE

A sample of faeces is sent to the laboratory for culture as soon as possible. This is not a particularly pleasant task because it means collecting some of the liquid faeces in a small pot, but it is the only way to tell if the stools are infected. By doing this the pathologist can identify the responsible organism.

BLOOD ANALYSIS

Both acute and chronic diarrhoea can upset the chemical balance of the blood. There is a danger of dehydration which can lead to a drop in blood pressure and eventually to kidney failure. Blood tests will show the extent of the dehydration. It will also reveal whether the person is anaemic, which can indicate a more serious underlying cause of the diarrhoea. A blood culture may also reveal any nasty organism which has infected the gut.

SIGMOIDOSCOPY

This is a direct examination of the lowermost part of the bowel using a flexible tube passed up through the anus. Provided stool culture and blood analysis have been performed and there has been no bleeding, sigmoidoscopy can be deferred for the first few days of an acute diarrhoeal illness. There is also no urgency for this test if the patient's condition improves. Very few general practitioners are trained to carry out such an investigation, so sigmoidoscopy is usually performed in the hospital outpatient department. Neither an anaesthetic, nor a stay in hospital are needed. A biopsy (the removal of a small piece of tissue for examination) may also be taken at this stage.

In Derek's case, both the initial blood and stool results were normal. I was concerned, however, that there might be a more serious cause for his symptoms (particularly as he had both weight loss and blood in the stools). I therefore referred him to the hospital as an emergency.

The sigmoidoscopy was carried out two days later and showed swelling and ulceration of the rectum (the lowermost part of the bowel, just above the anus). There were no signs of any tumours or cancer. The findings pointed towards an infection. Although E. Coli is the most common organism to cause diarrhoea, it does not affect the rectum, so this particular cause could be ruled out.

A biopsy of the lining of the rectum was taken and looked at under the microscope. It showed specific inflammation consistent with an organism called Cyclospora cayetanesis. The following day the pathologist telephoned me to say that further examination of the stool had revealed the parasite Giardia lamblia. Both of these nasty bugs are found in India, so it was the holiday that was responsible. Derek quickly improved with a course of antibiotics, although these had to be continued for three weeks to ensure complete eradication of the organisms.

Conventional treatment

HYDRATION

The effect of the fluid loss in diarrhoea should never be underestimated, especially when abroad in a hot country or even in a good English summer. When the diarrhoea is at its height, the intestinal muscles are so twitchy that faeces pass along the bowel too quickly, so there is no time for fluid to be reabsorbed. To make matters worse some bacteria actually cause water to be excreted into the intestine from the bloodstream. Both of these factors result in large fluid and electrolyte losses.

Initial management should therefore focus on minimising the patient's dehydration. Where the loss of fluid is not severe, simply increasing the intake of water, is all that is necessary. It is also advantageous to combine water with glucose to maintain energy levels. Oral rehydration solutions have also been developed which simultaneously provide water, sodium, glucose and sometimes amino acids. These solutions mimic the composition of the fluid that is lost in diarrhoea. They can be obtained on prescription and from the chemist's. They are particularly useful in infants or patients with severe illnesses, who are liable to become dangerously dehydrated.

ANTIDIARRHOEAL DRUGS

These are useful for controlling symptoms in adults and older children.

- The most well known is Kaolin et Morph. The kaolin is designed to soak up the fluid and the morphine to reduce peristalsis in the intestines. However, it is now generally accepted that kaolin has little clinical effect and there is too little morphine in the mixture to do any good.

- Loperamide (trade name Imodium) works directly on the gut, slowing the passage of faeces through the intestines. In my experience, it generally produces excellent results, in most cases.
- Codeine reduces intestinal motility and may also cause sedation. While it is not as effective as loperamide, it does ease the cramp-like pains that often accompany loose motions. A combination of loperamide and codeine may produce better results than using them on their own.

ANTIBIOTICS

Empirical treatment of infective diarrhoea, either in the first instance, or when the stool culture is negative, remains controversial. However, there is increasing evidence that such treatment is effective in reducing the duration and severity of the illness, especially where diarrhoea is contracted by those travelling abroad. Two commonly prescribed antibiotics are Trimethoprim and Ciprofloxacin, a newer antibiotic and the drug of choice for infections from Africa and Asia. Usually a three day course of these agents is sufficient, although, on occasions, extended courses (up to three weeks) may be necessary where organisms, such as Cyclospora (which burrows into the gut wall), take longer to be eradicated.

Management of diarrhoea in children

This problem causes more worry to parents than virtually any other. Mild diarrhoea should be treated with adequate fluid replacement. It is not necessary to force children to eat over the first few days if they don't feel like it. Any weight they lose will be quickly made up when they start eating again.

Children have a lower threshold as far as the loss of certain chemicals from the body is concerned, particularly sodium. They also tend to lose fluid more rapidly than adults. If diarrhoea is severe, oral rehydration fluids (usually Dioralyte or Rehydrat) should be given. These are often flavoured to make them more palatable, although it may still be difficult to make the child take them.

> *Jamie was a nine week old baby who I visited at home. His mother said he had developed diarrhoea two days previously. She had stopped giving him milk and was trying to make him take boiled water. On examination, he didn't look well. However, his hydration level was reasonably good, so there was no immediate danger. In my experience babies do not like boiled water, so I encourage the mother to continue normal feeding whenever possible. Breast-feeding has in fact been shown to boost the immune system, which is vital in fighting off illness. In addition, a cessation of breast-feeding may lead to a reduction in the mother's milk supply. Jamie was able to take in a reasonably good supply of milk. Although it was less than normal, it was sufficient to maintain an adequate level of hydration. His diarrhoea settled naturally in a couple of days.*

The use of antidiarrhoeal agents is not recommended in children and may be harmful as it allows the bug to be in contact with the lining of the gut for longer periods. If the child continues to pass large amounts of liquid stool and is showing increasing lethargy and drowsiness, then hospital admission may be needed.

Alternative therapies

NATUROPATHY

While babies should continue to feed whenever possible, in adults, however, food should generally be withheld for twenty four hours (most causes of diarrhoea produce a loss of appetite in any case). During this time, only mineral water, apple juice or a salt and sugar solution (one tumbler of water to one spoonful of sugar and a pinch of salt) should be taken. As the diarrhoea subsides, liquid food with a high nutritional value should be introduced, for example boiled rice, vegetable juice or soups. Live yoghurt will help the intestine to return to its normal state, regenerating the protective anti-infective flora. This is particularly useful in cases of antibiotic-induced diarrhoea. Solid foods should then be started: boiled rice and steamed carrots, followed by bananas, hard boiled eggs and dried toast. The diet slowly returns to normal over the following few days.

A general multivitamin and high doses of vitamin C (1000 mg twice daily) should be taken to boost the body's own natural defences.

When abroad on holiday, scrupulous hygiene should be maintained. Don't forget to avoid tap water, ice cubes, raw food, salad, ice cream and any food from a cold buffet which also displays undercooked meat.

HOMOEOPATHY

In cases of both acute and chronic diarrhoea, homoeopathic preparations offer an effective alternative to orthodox drugs. Nevertheless, the choice of preparation is vital. As always, for a homoeopathic remedy to be successful, it is necessary to consider the person as a whole. However, some of the important, general properties of each remedy are discussed below. All are taken in the 6c potency unless otherwise indicated.

- **Aloe** This remedy is useful in those who are suffering from acute diarrhoea. This may be associated with flatulence, cold chills and a lack of appetite. The patient's tongue may also become red towards the tip. Stools are generally yellowish-green in colour. Aloe should be taken every half an hour, for ten doses, and then four times daily.
- **Aconite** This is particularly effective in treating diarrhoea that comes on very suddenly after a shock, exposure to cold wind, or overheating in summer. In these cases the abdomen is distended, and the person feels better after passing a stool. The 30c concentration should be taken if possible.
- **Argentum nit** This is the best remedy for diarrhoea associated with anxiety and apprehension, belching and a craving for salt or sweet things.
- **Arsenicum** This is successfully used for scanty, odourless, brown stools which seem to burn the skin around the anus, especially after cold drinks, ice cream or ripe fruit. Hot drinks may be soothing. Typically, the person who benefits most from this remedy is anxious, pale and thin.
- **China** Where the stools resemble chopped eggs and there is a great amount of wind, which is made worse by eating fruit. It is best for irritable people.

- **Colocynth** This is most suitable for diarrhoea accompanied by spasmodic, griping pains which may cause the person to double up. Pressure on the abdomen lessens the discomfort. The stools are copious, thin, frothy and yellowish in colour. Attacks are brought on by anger.
- **Dulcamara** Diarrhoea which comes on in damp weather or as a result of getting chilled after exertion, is best treated with this remedy. The stools are slimy, green and often streaked with blood. It is typically suited to calm, unworried personalities.
- **Phosphoric acid** This remedy is most useful for profuse, watery stools with particles of food in them. Relief occurs after a bowel movement. It should be used by bright, sensitive individuals.
- **Podophyllum** This is recommended where there are copious and offensive-smelling stools, which are the colour of pea soup and the consistency of batter. A great deal of wind and colic may also be experienced, together with a tremendous urge to open the bowels in the morning, which is followed by an empty feeling.
- **Pulsatilla** Diarrhoea which is worse at night and after cold drinks, onions and rich, fatty, foods have been consumed, responds well to this preparation. No two stools look alike. This remedy is appropriate for fair-haired, shy and gentle people, who gain weight easily.
- **Sulphur** In cases where this remedy is recommended, the need to pass a stool may propel the person out of bed around 5 a.m.! The anus feels hot and piles may be present. The faeces are yellow and offensive-smelling. Typically, the person who responds best to sulphur is an active, well-fed, lover of life.
- **Veratrum** This is best for profuse stools, accompanied by vomiting. The forehead may also break out into a cold sweat. Sufferers frequently crave iced water. This remedy is most suited to confident types.

As you can see, there are plenty of remedies to choose from. The nearer you get to finding your own symptoms in the list above, the more effective the treatment will be. However, I find I nearly always use one of the following:

- Aloe;
- Argentum nit;
- Arsenicum album;
- Sulphur
- Pulsatilla

HERBAL MEDICINE

- **Agrimony** This has a tremendous healing effect on the lining of the gut, quickly clearing diarrhoea and colic. It has been used since Saxon times for this purpose. Surprisingly, it was also the prime ingredient of *arquebusade water*, a battlefield remedy for gunshot wounds. Agrimony is taken as an infusion of the leaves of the herb, which are gathered before, and during, early flowering in summer. If fresh leaves are not available, then it can also be obtained in powdered form from your local health food shop. In this case, the infusion is made from two tablespoons of powder in a pint of water. This is heated gently (but not boiled) for ten minutes, strained and drunk by the cupful. The taste is pleasant and it is safe for children. As it passes into breast milk, it can also be taken by breast-feeding mothers whose babies are suffering from the condition. It is also possible to combine it with other soothing herbs, such as chamomile, marshmallow root, meadowsweet or ribwort plantain.
- **Geranium** This is its common name but it is officially known as American cranesbill. It is drunk as a tincture, taken either from the roots or stems (2 to 3 mls of the tincture, up to three times daily).
- **Tormentil** This contains up to twenty per cent tannins and is an excellent astringent. It is taken as a tincture (made from the herb's roots) in a dose of 2 mls, three times daily.
- **Garlic** This has been used in herbal medicine for over five thousand years and is an excellent natural antibiotic. The cloves are the active part of the plant – the dreadful odour is due to their high sulphur content. While the natural clove, when chewed, is marginally more effective than the deodorised preparations, I urge you not to inflict the smell on your family, friends or workmates!

ACUPUNCTURE

Both these alternative methods of treatment are effective for the relief of diarrhoea.

In diarrhoea, an upset in the flow of energy occurs along the stomach and spleen channels. Needles are placed at specific acupuncture points along each channel. The points used (see Figure 11.1) are:

- **Stomach 44** In the web, at the base of the second and third toes;
- **Stomach 39** Below the knee on the front of the leg, 9 cun below the lower border of the knee cap;
- **Stomach 35** 2 cun to the side of the navel;
- **Spleen 3** Located just behind the base of the big toe, where the spleen channel begins;
- **Spleen 14** 3 cun to the side of the umbilicus and 1 cun vertically downwards.

Measurements are in cun which is approximately the width of an index finger.

The needles are then stimulated for about twenty minutes. In my experience, the healing effect is enhanced by warmth. To heat the needles, dried moxa (derived from the mugwort herb *Artemisia vulgaris*) is used. The end of each needle is wrapped in a small amount of the herb and set alight. There is no risk of being burnt, as the moxa generates a moderate heat which is taken down the needle straight into the acupuncture point, enhancing the flow of energy (*Chi*) along the relevant channel.

> *Helen, a thirty six year old housewife, came to my surgery with her fourth episode of diarrhoea in the past year. She had three very young children and seemed to catch the infections from them. She had found that orthodox drugs always had side-effects, the main one being an increase in the cramp-like pains in her abdomen. Helen had tried homoeopathy some years previously, but had not found it successful, so had little faith in that branch of alternative medicine (I suspected that she had not been prescribed the medication most suitable for her). I therefore suggested to Helen that we try acupuncture and, after reassurance that the needles would not hurt, she agreed. I inserted needles into both stomach and spleen channels, using points near their origin and others nearest to the intestines. Helen was amazed the needles were virtually painless.*
>
> *The next day, Helen phoned me at the surgery to say that her diarrhoea was much better. She could not, however, conceal the amazement in her voice. Many people, although they are quite happy to try acupuncture, do not really expect it to work for them and are often pleasantly surprised by the results.*

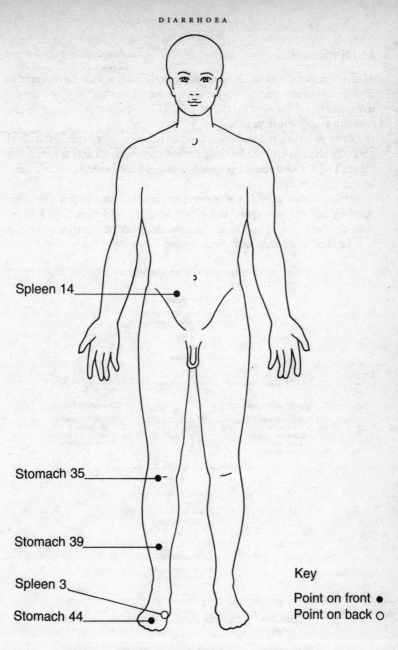

Figure 11.1 Acupuncture points for Diarrhoea

ACUPRESSURE

As the onset of diarrhoea is often acute and rapid, it may be difficult to arrange an acupuncture session at short notice. I teach all my patients the technique of acupressure for this reason. This is the use of massage on the relevant acupuncture points.

As the points in the abdomen tend to be too deep to rub manually, I generally recommend the following points: Stomach 39 and Spleen 3 (see Figure 11.1). These should be gently massaged for five minutes at a time, several times a day.

While it is not as effective as needling, acupressure can still give great relief. In fact, the next time I saw Helen, several months later, she told me that, despite being prone to the occasional attack of diarrhoea, she was able to clear it quickly with acupressure.

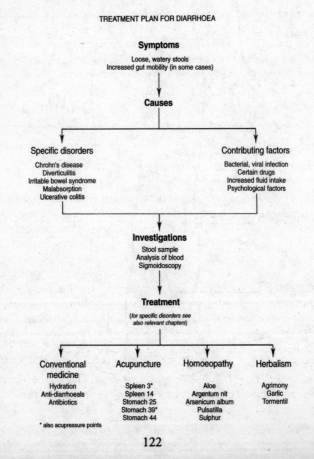

TREATMENT PLAN FOR DIARRHOEA

Symptoms

Loose, watery stools
Increased gut mobility (in some cases)

Causes

Specific disorders

Chrohn's disease
Diverticulitis
Irritable bowel syndrome
Malabsorption
Ulcerative colitis

Contributing factors

Bacterial, viral infection
Certain drugs
Increased fluid intake
Psychological factors

Investigations

Stool sample
Analysis of blood
Sigmoidoscopy

Treatment

*(for specific disorders see
also relevant chapters)*

Conventional medicine	Acupuncture	Homoeopathy	Herbalism
Hydration	Spleen 3*	Aloe	Agrimony
Anti-diarrhoeals	Spleen 14	Argentum nit	Garlic
Antibiotics	Stomach 25	Arsenicum album	Tormentil
	Stomach 39*	Pulsatilla	
	Stomach 44	Sulphur	

* also acupressure points

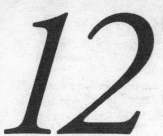

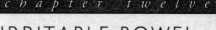

chapter twelve

IRRITABLE BOWEL SYNDROME

I rritable bowel syndrome (IBS), is the most common of all digestive disorders, estimated to affect one third of the population of Great Britain at some time in their lives, and one in six people on a regular basis. As a general practitioner, I meet patients with IBS every working day, so it is worth considering the condition in some detail.

What is IBS?

Most specialists now agree that IBS is not an actual disease but the way the intestinal muscle reacts to outside influences such as stress, infection and food. Faeces normally move along the large intestine by regular, smooth contraction of the muscles in the gut wall (peristalsis). In IBS, this contraction becomes irregular for some reason and can either be too strong or too weak. This produces a wide variety of symptoms, some of which mimic serious diseases such as bowel cancer and diverticulitis.

This presents the general practitioner with a difficult position, as it is essential to find any malignant tumours as quickly as possible. Thus, over half of all probable IBS cases are referred to the hospital outpatient department for tests. Unfortunately, a specific test does not exist which can prove a person is suffering from IBS. Often a diagnosis is made by process of elimination, if all other tests are normal. This is a time-consuming process and often increases patients' anxiety while they await the results.

Normal

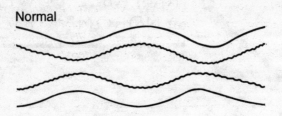

Increased (Diarrhoea)

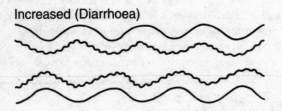

Decreased (Constipation)

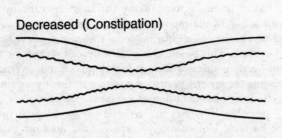

Figure 12.1   Peristalsis in IBS

I suspected that Jane, a forty seven year old woman, had developed diverticulitis (an inflammation of the large bowel which causes pain and diarrhoea). Jane had suffered these particular symptoms for nearly three weeks and the left side of her abdomen was acutely tender. I referred her urgently to a specialist at the hospital and she underwent quite rigorous tests, including an internal examination of the bowel with a sigmoidoscope, and a barium enema. As all the tests were normal, a diagnosis of Irritable Bowel Syndrome was made.

What causes IBS?

The majority of people can trace their IBS back to a significant event:

- An attack of gastro-enteritis which makes the intestines over reactive and sensitive;
- A course of antibiotics, particularly if longer than five days, which alters the delicate balance of helpful bacteria in the gut;
- A time of stress such as divorce, the threat of redundancy, bereavement, exams or financial worries;
- Certain foods may aggravate the condition;
- The regular use of laxatives undoubtedly irritates the bowel. The majority of the population of the West, seem to be under the mistaken belief that daily emptying of the bowels is essential for good health. This is not necessarily the case (see Chapter 10).

While these are generally accepted as the main precipitating factors in IBS, it is not known why the condition affects some people and not others. However, it appears you are unlikely to develop IBS if you eat the sort of diet that does not upset you, avoid laxatives and learn to reduce, or at least cope with, the worries you have.

Who suffers with IBS?

It can occur at any age and in both sexes, although it is most common in people who are in their thirties and forties. The degree of severity can vary significantly. At one end of the spectrum are those people who only have mild symptoms. Although they may suffer symptoms from time to time, they do not consult a doctor as they do not feel IBS upsets their lives in any way. At the other, are those for whom IBS is devastating. In between the mild and the severe cases, are the great majority who manage quite well most of the time but still have to watch what they eat, as they find their gut plays up if they become tense or agitated.

What are the symptoms of IBS?

The main symptom is a disturbance of bowel habit, with or without abdominal pain. This sounds simple enough, however even these symptoms can present themselves in a number of different ways. Patients suffering from IBS can experience any combination of the following:

- Abdominal pain, usually low on the left side although it is occasionally to the right or centre of the abdomen;
- Diarrhoea, with or without pain;
- Constipation, usually with stomach pain. Stools are characteristically small and lumpy;
- Alternating diarrhoea and constipation, usually in an erratic fashion;
- An abdomen that feels bloated, distended and full of wind;
- Mucus in the stools or passed on its own.

This grouping of symptoms only occurs in IBS, whereas other conditions produce only one or two. The problem is, however, that the signs are not constant and vary widely between different patients. They may also differ in individual people at different times. Symptoms worsen during times of stress but may disappear at other times.

Lynne, *a thirty year old housewife, was one such person who developed bowel problems following the death of her mother. Her major symptoms included persistent diarrhoea, with tenesmus (a constant desire to open the bowels), a continuous passing of mucus and severe, low abdominal pain, on her left side. Her stomach always felt distended with wind. In addition to these physical symptoms, she felt isolated, panicky and was totally lacking in self confidence. Lynne's social life was ruined, her diet horribly restricted and she was constantly worried that her ill health would cause the breakdown of her marriage.*

Janet, *who was forty two, had similar symptoms to Lynne, but nothing like as severe. A sales representative, she had to report her figures to the board of the company every three months. Janet found this very stressful and always developed diarrhoea, pain and bloating in the couple of weeks leading up to these meetings. In between, her stomach would feel quite settled.*

Jack, *a thirty eight year old accountant, had recently been under pressure, both at work and at home. At the end of each tax year he found his volume of work greatly increased. At home, the eldest of his five children, a teenager, caused him constant worry because of his attitude to school. Over two years, Jack suffered increasing constipation, a distended abdomen and his faeces were like little pellets. He noticed that these symptoms were much worse when he became upset or worried.*

These three cases illustrate two very different types of Irritable Bowel Syndrome. The first type occurs where the intestine becomes twitchy and overactive, leading to diarrhoea and pain. Lynne and Janet fit into this group. The second type of IBS is where the gut is underactive, producing constipation and obvious abdominal distension, as in Jack's case. Most people have one or other of these two types, although symptoms may merge to produce alternating constipation and diarrhoea.

What is particularly confusing about IBS is that it can also produce a constellation of seemingly unassociated symptoms, including passing urine more frequently, back pain, insomnia, headaches, reduced sex drive, painful periods and often mild depression. It was not surprising, therefore, that doctors used to think IBS was a nervous disorder and that most sufferers were hypochondriacs, given the seemingly random symptoms. However, these symptoms are now recognised as an integral part of IBS.

As we have seen, IBS is not a simple diagnosis to make. Some patients may feel they are told they have Irritable Bowel Syndrome, merely to give them a label. Investigations are essential, for this reason.

Lynne's *symptoms were typical of IBS, so I was very definite in my diagnosis at the first consultation.*

Janet's *case was not so clear-cut. I told her I believed she was suffering from IBS and that investigations were necessary to exclude other conditions.*

Jack *was worried about cancer. Although I was almost sure he had IBS, I arranged a barium enema to exclude the possibility of a tumour. The fear of cancer is very understandable in anyone with long standing bowel problems. The sufferer will often be greatly reassured by investigations. Jack's tests were completely normal. This, in itself, produced an improvement in his symptoms, by removing a source of worry.*

The four cardinal symptoms

As IBS sufferers have at least one of the four cardinal symptoms (pain, diarrhoea, constipation and wind) it is worth looking at these in greater detail.

DO YOU HAVE ABDOMINAL PAIN?

Pain in the gut drives most people with IBS to see their doctor. It is usually on the lower left side but can actually occur anywhere in the abdomen. It is occasionally referred to more distant areas of the body such as the tip of the shoulder. The pain may range from a dull ache to sheer agony, which may cause the sufferer to double up. It tends to come and go in waves, building up to a crescendo and then falling away again particularly after meals. The pain is only relieved by passing wind or opening the bowels.

DO YOU HAVE DIARRHOEA?

In IBS, diarrhoea may occur on its own, alternate with constipation and occur with, or without, mucus. A common scenario is a period of constipation, followed by a sudden attack of diarrhoea. This type of diarrhoea is different from the infective type where large quantities of watery motions are passed. In IBS, the quantity of faeces is much the same as any healthy person's, though more frequent and sloppy. It is usually worse in the morning and gradually settles during the day. The associated pain may be relieved by opening the bowels. Some have to get up at night for a bowel movement, others do not have their sleep disturbed.

Research has shown that sixty per cent of IBS sufferers with diarrhoea, have an intolerance to one, or more, foods. In addition, this type of IBS afflicts those people who are generally more anxious than those who experience the constipation IBS.

DO YOU HAVE CONSTIPATION?

The symptoms of IBS are much more common in people who have suffered long-standing constipation. A very important sign of IBS is where the patient complains of constipation but has frequent bowel movements (they feel their bowels have not been emptied completely).

DO YOU HAVE WIND?

IBS sufferers do not produce excessive wind. It is simply that the motility of their gut is abnormal and gas is often unable to escape, building up inside the intestine. This eventually causes the abdomen to distend and become very painful. Belching or the passing of wind can be most embarrassing but at least it helps to relieve the distension.

Diagnosis

There is no doubt that IBS represents a diagnostic problem because of the wide range of symptoms it produces. The traditional solution (as stated previously) is to refer the person to hospital for investigation. Knowledge of the syndrome has now sufficiently increased to enable the general practitioner to diagnose the condition in the practice.

The patient may well be able to diagnose the condition on his or her own. Referral of patients to hospital is strictly necessary, however, for those with weight loss, rectal bleeding or gross faecal impaction.

HISTORY

A careful and detailed history is of paramount importance in order to diagnose IBS. Questions are asked about symptoms of pain, weight gain or loss, bowel function changes, abdominal distension and potential precipitating factors such as foods, drugs, stress and lifestyle changes.

A study which compared the incidence of twenty abdominal symptoms thought to be common in IBS, in two groups of patients (one diagnosed with IBS and the other, with organic abdominal disease), showed that there were eight symptoms that were far more common in patients with IBS:

- Abdominal pain;
- Diarrhoea and/or constipation;
- Pain relieved by defaecation;
- Frequent bowel movements;
- Loose bowel movements with the onset of the pain;
- Abdominal distension;
- Passage of mucus;
- A sensation of incomplete emptying of the rectum.

It is uncommon for IBS sufferers to have all these symptoms but, if they have at least four, then in my mind there is no doubt of the diagnosis. They will have other problems relating to their IBS which may confuse the issue so I always question them directly about these eight symptoms.

EXAMINATION

IBS is virtually always diagnosed from the case history and any abnormal findings on examination merely help to confirm the diagnosis. The only real value is to exclude signs of organic disease such as anaemia and weight loss, which militate against a diagnosis of IBS.

Graham had five positive IBS features. There was little doubt, therefore, that he had IBS but he was concerned about the persistence of his symptoms and felt that they should be investigated.

On examination, Graham was tender over the bowel on the left side of the abdomen, along the course of the intestine. This is the one positive sign of IBS that may be found on external palpation. A rectal examination (where a finger is gently pushed through the anus to feel for any tumours that might be causing constipation) revealed that Graham had no lumps but was tender. I could also feel the hard bullet-like faeces which are so typical of IBS.

Sigmoidoscopy is a procedure which enables the colon to be viewed directly. In IBS, the bowel generally appears normal, however there are certain positive findings which may help to confirm IBS: obvious spasm or hypermotility of the bowel (the procedure itself may provoke the symptoms), a slight swelling of the bowel lining (especially in IBS sufferers who have diarrhoea) and excess mucus secretion (giving the intestines a lustrous appearance).

Management of IBS

Although IBS is not fatal, it is a chronic, relapsing disorder and causes much suffering. It is distressing and inconvenient. The management and treatment strategy depend to a large extent on the doctor's view of the relative importance of the constitutional, psychological and dietary factors in the individual patient.

REASSURANCE AND EXPLANATION

For all my patients, I start treatment with a careful explanation of the symptoms and emphasize the benign nature of the condition as many patients think they may have a serious disease. Treatment of IBS really starts during the discussion of the patient's history and their examination. Asking questions about their diet, stress and emotional state enables the doctor to isolate possible contributing factors. Counselling alone can often produce an improvement in many IBS sufferers.

Conventional treatment

In treating IBS doctors prescribe three types of drug:

- **Antispasmodics** These make the bowel relax and relieve the colicky spasm that causes so much pain. They appear to have no serious side-effects, although they may impair driving ability or raise blood pressure. Examples of this type of drug include Colofac and Motilium;
- **Bulk laxatives** These are usually based on the drug ispaghula (Fybogel). This makes the stools soft, bulky and easy to pass. They also do not have any significant side-effects;
- **Mild antidepressants** These are designed to relieve the stress and anxiety that is associated with IBS. Unfortunately, they usually have side-effects. It is not advisable to continue long-term use of drugs, which affect the mind. Although in theory they should help, in practice many IBS sufferers do not find antidepressants to be of much value.

A combination of these medicines often gives relief over the short term. However, as IBS is often a long-term disorder, drugs cannot really be the permanent answer. If you can accept that what you eat, how you live and view life will probably have more effect on your bowel than anything else, then you are already halfway to coping with IBS. It should be your aim to take drugs for as short a period of time as possible. Once the bulk laxatives have produced a soft, formed motion every day, for a period of two weeks, then this should be maintained by a high-fibre diet.

Similarly, when the antispasmodics reduce the pain, then it is possible to take a fresh look at the tension which may be causing the bowel muscles to seize up. Realising you can improve your condition on your own, will lift your spirits and help you to take control of your own health.

Lynne, *who had severe IBS, had been taking the various drugs for some time and had found virtually no relief from them.*

Janet, *who had the milder form, didn't fancy taking any orthodox medication.*

Jack, *with the constipation type of IBS, had only tried a proprietary laxative from the chemist which had actually made him feel worse. All three were keen to help themselves to manage the disorder.*

Self-help

DIET

> ❛ I am convinced that my IBS is caused by some of the things I eat. If I ever have cereal for breakfast or a meal cooked with onions, then my stomach starts gurgling and before long, I am rushing to the toilet. ❜

Nearly three quarters of IBS sufferers have an intolerance to certain foodstuffs. Without doubt, some foods contain chemicals which upset the lining of the bowel and therefore aggravate the symptoms of IBS. Examples include: wheat, corn, dairy products, coffee, oats, rye, tea, citrus fruits, fatty and fried foods, onions, cabbage, salads and alcohol.

The most common of all these irritants is undoubtedly wheat which is present in many breakfast cereals. People who have an intolerance to wheat, usually experience the same with corn. Unfortunately, as wheat is in so many products, it is not easy to cut out of the diet. However, wholefood and health food shops sell products that do not contain wheat. These products are manufactured mainly for people with coeliac disease, who are unable to absorb the gluten in wheat. A wide range of products is now available including wheat-free bread, flour, biscuits and pasta. Many of these are available on prescription.

Dairy products are the next most frequent cause of food intolerance. This category includes milk, butter, cheese and yoghurt, but you should also watch out for processed and packet foods which may contain them. Look carefully at the list of ingredients on packets of biscuits, margarine, cereals, puddings, sauces and sweets, as you may find whey, whey solids, milk solids and skimmed milk powder are included, all of which come from milk. Milk contains a sugar called lactose, which is broken down in the gut by an enzyme called lactase. Some people don't produce enough lactase, so can't break down the lactose in milk products properly. This is particularly common in those IBS sufferers who have diarrhoea.

Lynne *felt her bowels were sensitive to so many foods that she was never able to eat out at friends' houses or to go to restaurants. Even the thought of going on holiday did not appeal to her. Her mealtimes had become totally dominated by her IBS. Most people are not as sensitive to as many foods as they think. If you are worried that a particular food may upset you (especially when you are eating out), then a level of anxiety is* *generated, causing the disruption of the digestive process and the unpleasant IBS symptoms. Lynne was quite happy to agree with this suggestion as she knew she became very tense while eating out, anticipating how her bowels would react.*

*When **Janet** said her IBS was made worse by eating breakfast, it could have been due to the wheat in the cereal, or to the milk she poured on to it. It could even have been caused by the cup of coffee she had with her breakfast!*

***Jack** found that his IBS would flare up if he ate a large amount of dairy produce, particularly cheese. However, small portions did not seem to affect him. In cases such as these, the solution is to cut the offending food from the diet for a while, allowing the body to become accustomed to being without it. Thereafter the food should be eaten occasionally or in small quantities. Once Jack accepted that a certain amount of cheese did not cause an adverse reaction, then his level of anxiety fell and he was able to eat more cheese than he thought would be possible.*

It may be obvious which food disagrees with you, but if you are not sure, try this simple regime, for two weeks:

- Cut out all red meat, fatty foods, fried foods, coffee and alcohol completely;
- Have as little dairy produce as you find possible;
- Have a simple, leisurely breakfast of fruit juice, cereal and wholemeal toast with vegetable margarine and marmalade or honey;
- For lunch, have wholemeal bread sandwiches or salad and fresh fruit;
- In the evening, try a vegetarian dish, fish or chicken with salad or fresh vegetables, followed by fresh fruit;
- Drink as little tea or coffee as possible and cut out alcohol initially for about two to three weeks;
- Banish smoking from your life for ever.

If, over the two-week period, this regime makes you feel better, then try introducing some of the offending foods in small quantities, at the rate of one type every two days, noting any reactions these new foods provoke. You can then adjust your eating habits accordingly.

Lynne *found she was sensitive to wheat, dairy produce and red meat. I was sure that stress was also a significant contributing factor in her IBS.*

Janet *noticed an immediate improvement as soon as she left off cereal, milk and coffee for her breakfast. By reintroducing them individually, she noticed that her griping pains and diarrhoea were brought on by the cereal and coffee, indicating an intolerance to wheat and caffeine. Leaving these out of her daily diet, made a tremendous difference to her condition.*

Jack *had already discovered he was sensitive to dairy products, as he had found he was unable to eat too much cheese. In addition, red meat (mainly lamb and pork), white wine and lager all produced IBS symptoms when they were reintroduced into his diet. Surprisingly, red wine and bitter beer did not upset him.*

EXERCISE

The majority of us in the West, take less exercise than our counterparts did twenty years ago. The reasons for this are varied and differ for each person but, in general, lifestyles have become more convenience-orientated. Lifts and escalators are everywhere and at airports, we would rather stand on moving walkways, than push trolleys ourselves. Many families now have two cars and use them for every little thing. If children live more than two hundred yards from their school, then walking is out of the question. Leisure time tends to be spent in front of the television, especially now that a vast array of programmes are available via satellite. With pollution at an all time high, nipping out for a quick walk is not as enjoyable, as roads are becoming more and more congested. Even going out to the country for an afternoon's hiking, is not as tempting is it once was.

Our body muscles thrive on exercise and those in our intestines are no exception. The more you work, the stronger and fitter they become. Research has proved that nearly all people with IBS show a marked improvement with regular exercise. In addition, becoming fit makes you feel much more lively and energetic and this undoubtedly helps you to relax and lower stress levels.

Whichever sport you choose, it is vital that you find it enjoyable. Although it may be unpopular with some people, jogging is an excellent form of exertion, for example. If you are able to take up a team sport, play with a friend or join a group activity, you'll find it is much easier to get fit. It is harder to motivate yourself on your own. Where work commitments make team sport impossible, other alternatives such as swimming, cycling and walking with friends, or on your own, may be equally enjoyable.

Stress

Stress is absolutely not a sign of weakness. Why is it so many of us feel ashamed and defensive at having a condition that may be caused by stress? It is quite illogical. The patients I see in my surgery are not apologetic about having coronary heart disease, high blood pressure, colitis or asthma. Those who suffer from stress-related conditions, however, react quite differently. In the past, stress was considered as a sign of weakness in our society but thankfully this is gradually changing. Today, although many people are still reluctant to admit to stress, at least a growing number are beginning to realise the harmful effects it can have on the body.

Can you remember the stressful times in your lives? Perhaps it was long ago, when you were called to see the head teacher? Or when you were waiting for your first job interview? Perhaps it was before an important sports match or taking part in a play? Can you recall the 'butterflies' in your stomach? You may even have experienced diarrhoea or complete loss of appetite. All of us notice a connection between how our insides are linked with fear, emotion and anxiety.

WHAT DOES STRESS DO TO OUR BODY?

Stress has two main effects. Firstly it stimulates the adrenal glands to produce adrenalin which makes our hearts beat faster, our blood pressure rise and the muscles in our intestines contract. This is known as the 'adrenalin surge' and is common in sports people before a big event.

The production of adrenalin as a result of stress can be beneficial over a short period of time. Unfortunately, it can be destructive to our body systems over a long period of time. As well as producing adrenalin, the adrenal glands are responsible for releasing other hormones which boost the immune system. Constant stress (especially as a result of worrying), reduces this hormone output. This is why many people, after periods of stress, get colds, feel run down, tired, have aches and pains or develop digestive disorders (particularly IBS).

DOES STRESS CAUSE IRRITABLE BOWEL SYNDROME?

Most sufferers of IBS can trace the onset of their symptoms to some stressful event (such as exams, marital problems, financial difficulties or bereavement). Young adults generally develop IBS because they find life stressful. Tests have shown that a distressed mind leads to an overactive bowel. It has not yet been discovered whether IBS patients react differently from other people or whether they simply have a particularly sensitive colon. It appears the digestive systems of those who do not have IBS, become less disturbed the longer the stress continues, which would indicate that, in IBS, the sufferer fails to adapt in this way. As it is common for people to eat and drink more when life gets tough, these factors may also have a part to play in IBS.

In people who have IBS, when stress levels are high, the bowel contracts more than in non-sufferers. This causes pain, which produces more stress, creating a vicious circle:

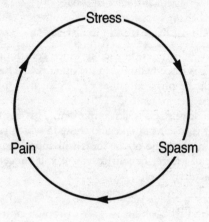

CAN'T I JUST TAKE A TABLET?

There is not much point in taking medicines if you don't tackle the underlying problem – in this case stress. A few people cannot accept their irritable bowel is connected in any way to their personality, their way of life or their anxiety. They prefer to think it is entirely a physical disease, which they can leave safely in the hands of their doctor. They wrongly believe a prescription is all they need to be well. Sadly for these people, the symptoms of IBS are unlikely to improve.

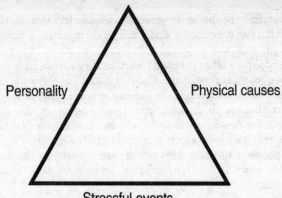

SO WHAT CAN I DO ABOUT STRESS?

The diagram above illustrates the factors which contribute to IBS. Each side of the triangle is directly linked to the other two. The ways in which you can deal with the physical causes of IBS, such as food intolerance, have been covered (see pages 133–135).

The management of stress is also important. This can be divided into the measures you yourself can take and those in which you will initially need medical help. As some of the ideas will appeal to you more than others, it will be of greater benefit to you if you concentrate on those which seem particularly useful.

SELF-HELP IN STRESS

Start by learning to recognise the signs of stress in yourself:

- Do you sit on the edge of the chair, tap your fingers, bang your knees together or clench your fists?
- Do you suffer with headaches, neck aches or back pain?
- Do you feel restless?

All of us suffer from stress to some degree and it manifests itself in different ways. In people with IBS, once it reaches a certain level it triggers off the symptoms. This level will vary from person to person, but it is essential to recognise it and to keep stress below the level that triggers IBS for you.

THE ANTI-STRESS PLAN

There are a bewildering number of ways of relieving stress, many c which are described in magazines. Unfortunately, most are difficult t stick to for any length of time. I have devised a ten point plan which have recommended to many of my patients and have fine-tuned it ove the years. A few changes to your lifestyle are involved, however man people have commented on how easy it is to follow, and stick to, th plan.

- **STEP 1** Write down the situations that give you most trouble, that you dread most and that you get most anxious about. Then note if your bowel becomes irritable during these situations. Nex imagine each of these situations in turn, and visualise yourself as pleasantly relaxed. Lower your shoulders, unclench your fists and breathe deeply and evenly, until you are able to think about that situation without anxiety.

- **STEP 2** As you sit at your desk, kitchen table, in the car, bus or train, develop the habit of noticing muscle tension – particularly in the feet, thighs, hands, shoulders, neck, mouth and forehead. Then relax them by alternately tightening and loosening each set of muscles. You may already put aside some time to relax in the peace and quiet at home, but it is vitally important to be able to do this at any time.

- **STEP 3** At first, learn to prioritise, both at work and in your personal life. Do you really need all that overtime money? Do yoι really need to bring that work home? Is it really necessary to tidγ the bedrooms every day? Must you go out to the neighbour's jewellery party or is your time better spent with your family? Always bear in mind that more stress is caused by things which are left undone, than by those that are finished. Remember that only a certain number of tasks can be performed in a day. Doing the small repairs in the house first, for example, will bring a grea sense of achievement. You will then be free to tackle other jobs.

- **STEP 4** Reduce any major tasks to manageable components and plan your time effectively. You may find it helps to divide each day's tasks into priority categories, such as A, B, and C. Start witl the ones marked A and only attempt B and C if you have time. If you run out of time, leave them and do not feel guilty. They are the least important and can wait.

- **STEP 5** Learn to delegate. Stressed people often try to do everything themselves. When your work load is heavy ask your staff (if you have people working under you) or colleagues to help out, and let them get on with it. At home, make sure the chores are shared and don't keep checking if they have been done. Even if a job is not carried out as well, or as quickly, as you would have done it, does it really matter all that much?

The first five steps are mainly organisational. The next five are concerned with enjoying life and your free time:

- **STEP 6** Develop a hobby or interest that is relaxing and non-competitive. Make sure it is something you really like doing and don't worry what other people think. If you can't think of anything, buy some magazines and explore the different possibilities.
- **STEP 7** Take regular exercise. It lifts the spirits, works off the pent-up tension which wears you down, revives your outlook on life and gives you more energy, making it far easier to cope with stress. Swimming, cycling, jogging and brisk walking are excellent. If you prefer a competitive sport such as squash, make sure you don't worry about your place on the league ladder!
- **STEP 8** Review your friends. As the years pass, it may be that you need to develop new ones. Friends should make us feel good and increase our self-esteem. It may well be that your current friends undermine your confidence or talk about themselves all the time.
- **STEP 9** Love is understanding rather than criticizing. Giving and receiving love is a sign of strength not weakness. If you show affection to family and friends, they will give it back. There is nothing like someone showing they love you to boost your morale.
- **STEP 10** Plan to do something you enjoy every day and then make sure you do it. It doesn't have to be anything major – a hot bath, your favourite television programme, a walk in the country or a relaxing glass of wine. Keep remembering through the day that there is still that pleasure to come.

When I give my patients a copy of this plan, I can see they are thinking, 'Here's something else which is good in theory, but not in practice.'

However, most come back telling me how it has changed their lives, lowered their stress levels and, most importantly, greatly improved their IBS symptoms.

Lynne's IBS had started shortly after her mother's death. The death of a loved one is one of life's most stressful events. Apart from the grief and the huge gap that was left in Lynne's life, other problems had developed: there was no one to help her look after the children and her daughter Jane started misbehaving at school; Lynne's husband was struggling with his job and there was no guarantee of a steady income each month.

I encouraged Lynne to follow the anti-stress plan; she wrote down her main stresses. Simply recognising these problem areas made her feel calmer and more determined to do something about the situation.

Lynne started learning to relax as often as possible and exercised to loosen the tension in her muscles. She even bought some gym equipment to use at home. She had never had the courage to do this before, as she had previously thought it unladylike to lump weights about. She prioritised, setting herself achievable tasks each day, not always aiming to have the house looking perfect, and leaving the ironing if she felt too tired. Changing her friends made a big difference to her life. Lynne tactfully stopped seeing the ones who made her feel depressed and developed friendships with other people who really took an interest in her. It took a while, but her social life has now changed completely. Finally, she makes sure every day is varied, and she looks forward to doing something enjoyable. As she had always been interested in tapestry, she joined a local class twice a week. One day, she rents a video, and another, has lunch with a friend.

These were all simple changes but have made Lynne's life much more relaxed and in fact showed that her IBS could be improved by her own actions. Both Janet and Jack also used this plan to great effect.

HOW CAN I COPE WITH A MAJOR STRESSFUL EVENT?

The plan above will help you to deal with day to day stress. Stronger measures may be needed for specific events such as bereavement, divorce, personal injury or illness, dismissal from work, new job or change in financial state. For stressful events such as these, the use of self-hypnosis can be very helpful.

Hypnosis
This simply induces a very pleasant state of relaxation (particularly beneficial in any case of IBS where stress is the main factor). While you are in a 'trance', the therapist will work with you to clear the subconscious feelings that inevitably arise as a result of major stressful events.

As well as working on the stress that makes your IBS worse, the hypnotherapist will also spend time suggesting ways to control the symptoms. A simple way is to imagine you have a hot water bottle on your abdomen and learn to relate the sensation of warmth to gaining control over your gut.

For Lynne, it was coping with the death of her mother which, although it occurred two years ago, was still just as painful. Lynne felt very guilty, believing she should have shown more love to her mother and done more to help her. By working deeply on these feelings, the therapist was able to remove the extreme feelings of guilt she was experiencing. She had an excellent response to hypnosis and by practising it herself at home she finally gained control over her IBS.

CAN I CHANGE MY PERSONALITY?

The third leg of the triangle (see page 138) is our personality. Have you ever wondered whether there might be a connection between your irritable bowel and the type of person you are? It has long been recognised by doctors that certain diseases are often found in people with certain types of personality. You may have talked yourself to other people with IBS and felt you had much in common.

It appears that people with IBS fit into one of two personality types:

- The first is the person who is very strong and forceful who has a burning desire to win at everything. If you fall into this first category, ask yourself whether being so competitive and in a constant state of tension, contributes to your irritable bowel. If so, you have to slow down and allow your adrenal glands to relax. Stop looking at your watch so often and decide you're only going to do one task at a time. Don't prepare the next day's notes, for example, while watching television, or mark homework while cooking the supper. Learn to lose occasionally – winning is not vital and you are only playing for the fun of the game itself after all.

- The second is the perfectionist who finds it hard to say 'No', and is seldom satisfied with their achievements. Other people take advantage of them and as they are so helpful and obliging, they always listen and shoulder everyone's problems. If you fall into this category, put time aside each day that is entirely for you. Use it to do whatever you want to do without feeling guilty about it. For some ideas see pages 139–41. Really enjoy yourself. Try learning to say 'No' which, although difficult at first, will slowly become easier. Imagine saying it at first, perhaps when you are lying in the bath, and think up a phrase that won't upset the person who requires something of you. Go over this several times until you are comfortable with the idea. Then, when the situation happens in real life, you will find it easier to say 'No'.

Changing your personality on a long-term basis is not easy, but it can be done!

Treatment of the four cardinal symptoms of IBS

So far we have dealt with changing the three factors that are closely linked to IBS (the food intolerance, stress and personality triangle on page 138). The lifestyle changes mentioned in the last few pages are the key to curing the bowel problem in the long term. However, inevitably these changes are gradual and slow to work. It is necessary, therefore, initially to take steps to relieve the major symptoms of pain, constipation, diarrhoea and wind. It is worth noting that many doctors and patients now favour alternative methods of treatment to drug therapy.

COPING WITH PAIN

Most irritable bowel sufferers have abdominal pain, which, in many cases, is very severe.

Conventional treatment
This is with painkillers and antispasmodics. They do not seem to be effective in the long term.

Naturopathy

Simple self-help measures on the other hand, seem to be beneficial. When pain strikes:

- Breathe deeply, concentrating on the passage of air through your nostrils and then exhale slowly;
- Make sure you do not tense up and try to keep your abdominal muscles relaxed all the time;
- Find a comfortable position where the pain is less severe. This may be lying on your back with your knees bent upwards, or it may be on your front with your legs straight;
- Use a hot compress, such as a towel or hot water bottle, applied to your lower abdomen;
- Be active: go for a walk or do some gentle stretching exercises. If you are in bed, or in a chair, then get up and walk around.

Herbal remedies

Which herb you choose depends very much on your individual preference. It will be virtually impossible to drink a herbal remedy regularly which has a nasty taste. Try a selection of the following and see which you prefer:

- Infuse 20 gm of hops in one litre of boiling water for ten minutes and drink a cupful after meals. Hops can be obtained either from a health food store or from a home brewing shop;
- Infuse 20 gm of lemon balm in the same way, and drink a cupful with meals;
- Heat a tablespoon of fennel seeds in a cup of milk, and drink while hot;
- Infuse 5 gm of lavender in a litre of boiling water, leave for five minutes, strain and drink three cups a day between meals;
- Infuse four leaves of mint in a cup of boiling water, leave for five minutes and drink twice daily. An infusion of fresh thyme can also be made in the same way.

You may also find it useful to cook with herbs which aid digestion, toning and soothing the gut. Such herbs include: cumin, fennel, garlic, marjoram, mint, parsley, rosemary, sage and thyme.

Homoeopathy

The choice of remedy depends on the nature of the pain. Seeing a qualified therapist is advisable, but you can also try taking one of the following remedies:

- **Nux vomica**: particularly where the pain is left-sided and relieved by opening the bowels;
- **Belladonna**: if the abdomen is distended and the sufferer feels better when doubled-up;
- **Colocynth**: when the sufferer cannot sit still and, again, feels better when doubled-up;
- **Magnesia phosphorica**: if the person feels better for applying heat to their abdomen.

The dose is two tablets at night and two in the morning, with extra tablets in the day if needed. Either 6c or 30c can be used.

Acupuncture

I usually reserve this for the severer cases of intractable pain, as it involves the expense of regular visits to a therapist. Having said this, it is very effective. By stimulating four or so needles, the acupuncturist will try to restore the imbalance in the stomach and large intestine channels. This involves inserting the needles at the appropriate points in the abdomen and feet. Acupuncture is fully discussed in Chapter 3.

DEALING WITH CONSTIPATION

Constipation occurs in roughly half of those suffering with IBS and arises as a direct result of reduced gut motility. The ways of relieving it are quite simple and should all be used together:

- Eat a high-fibre diet;
- Drink plenty of fluids, preferably warm and non-alcoholic. Aim for about three pints of fluid per day. Tannin in tea tends to constipate, so drink a herb tea instead. There are several, pleasant-tasting ones available, but if you find their taste a bit sharp, add some honey;
- Don't ignore the urge to open your bowels;
- Allow plenty of time for each bowel movement. Try getting up a few minutes early for breakfast to allow sufficient time for the rectum to empty completely;

- You may find it useful to infuse 5 gm of basil leaves or flowering tips in boiling water, straining the liquid before drinking;
- Carrot soup is also effective – simmer two lb of carrots in one pint of water for two hours, then blend in a liquidiser;
- Soak figs or prunes in water overnight. Figs can be eaten raw, but prunes should be cooked before eating;
- Take natural liquorice;
- Eat charcoal biscuits;
- Homoeopathic remedies such as Aesculus (where there is a sensation of fullness in the rectum after a motion) and Lycopodium (where there are rumblings in the bowels but no action) are particularly recommended.

AVOIDING LAXATIVES

When reading the advertisements for laxatives, it is easy to form the impression that not opening your bowels every day is something really serious. People end up using larger and larger quantities of ever-stronger laxatives, with less and less effect. They are afraid to stop taking them in case they become more constipated. There is, however, no known relationship between a daily bowel movement and good health. The problem with laxatives is they empty the whole of the large intestine and it takes several days before a normal quantity of stool to collect once again. During this time, you will not have another bowel movement as there is nothing in the bowel to pass. This leads you to believe you are constipated and to take more laxatives. In this way, your bowel is never given a chance to work normally. In IBS, where there is already a motility problem, this further increases the severity of the symptoms.

If you are already taking laxatives regularly, do not despair. If you cut them down slowly, your bowel will gradually regain its motility (although this can take several weeks).

MANAGING DIARRHOEA

Diarrhoea is one of the major symptoms of IBS and can be the most embarrassing and incapacitating of all. It occurs when the muscles in the intestines become overactive, passing the food along too quickly, for enough water to be absorbed (see pages 107–122). In IBS, diarrhoea is generally worse in the morning, gradually settling as the day goes on. The management of diarrhoea involves several steps:

- Strange as it may seem, the **high-fibre diet** which is recommended for constipation, may also work for those who suffer from diarrhoea, although it can initially make the stools rather sticky;
- **Bulking laxatives**, such as Fybogel, help to bind the loose stools together. It may seem contradictory to take bulking laxatives for diarrhoea, but they are often beneficial to IBS sufferers. Only the bulking type may be used, as the others irritate the bowel;
- **Anti-diarrhoea drugs** like codeine and Imodium can be of great benefit in the short term;
- **Homoeopathic remedies** for diarrhoea include Natrum Sol for looseness and cramps, Podophyllum for watery yellow stools in the morning, with a sensation of weakness in the rectum, and Sulphur for diarrhoea associated with excess wind.

Before any event that is worrying you could also try:

- one teaspoon of honey in one fluid ounce of hot water, stirring until the honey melts, then adding three drops of the essential oil of geranium, sipping it slowly;
- one dessertspoon of cider vinegar in a glass of water, to be drunk before each meal;
- one dessertspoon of arrowroot in a small quantity of water until smooth. Top this up with one pint of boiling water and drink when cool. It can be flavoured, if preferred, with blackcurrant juice.

MINIMISING WIND AND ABDOMINAL DISTENSION

Belching or passing wind can be most embarrassing, but at least it relieves the immediate problem. IBS sufferers do not produce excessive wind, it is simply that the motility of their gut is abnormal and gas is often unable to escape, building up inside the intestines. This eventually causes the abdomen to distend and become very painful.

For many, abdominal bloating is the worst symptom of all, as it is not only uncomfortable, but also makes shopping and wearing the latest fashions quite difficult. However, there are several methods of clearing wind and therefore relieving the distended stomach:

- Avoid constipation wherever possible. A blocked rectum prevents gas escaping so it has no alternative but to gather within the intestines;
- Be aware that you may be swallowing excess air as you eat or drink, so try to avoid this;
- You may find a low-fibre diet helpful; more peeled vegetables, fish, lean meat, white rice, bread and pasta;
- Try infusing the root or the leaves of angelica and drinking a cupful while hot, whenever necessary;
- Chew mustard seeds with plenty of water;
- Suck sweets containing oil of peppermint or put a few drops of peppermint essence in warm water and drink it slowly;
- Add a teaspoon of cinnamon or nutmeg to warm milk. You can sweeten this with honey and drink as required;
- Infuse any of the following in boiling water and drink when it has cooled slightly: marjoram, grated ginger root, fresh or dried basil leaves. All of these can also be sweetened with honey.

SUMMARY

Lynne *had severe IBS, which was completely destroying her life. She had previously depended on orthodox drugs, but it was only when she took a holistic approach to her condition, that her agony started to settle. Changing her diet, controlling her stress level and altering her personality required dedication and commitment, but the benefits were numerous. Lynne can now lead a normal life. From time to time she takes Nux vomica and an infusion of hops, to control any flare up in her symptoms while regularly using self-hypnosis to cope with the stress in her life.*

Janet, *who had the diarrhoea type of IBS, did not like taking conventional tablets but was able to cure her diarrhoea with a high-fibre diet, homoeopathic sulphur, fennel and arrowroot.*

Jack, *who experienced the constipation type, settled his problem mainly by reducing his stress level, changing his diet, taking regular exercise and using liquorice and homoeopathic Lycopodium.*

There is no wonder pill to cure IBS and until that day comes, relief of the condition is really down to you. There will be times when the condition goes away completely. When this happens, enjoy life and at the same time try to work out what has happened to settle your symptoms. If the

IBS comes back, then don't become depressed, just assess the changes you have made recently and consider whether you could have done things differently to keep the IBS at bay.

With all the present research into IBS, new discoveries will undoubtedly be made in the next few years. Perhaps it will be due to a physical defect in the body. Hopefully, simpler ways will be found to examine the bowel, making sigmoidoscopies a thing of the past. A simple, non-intrusive test may be developed, to permit doctors to make a firm diagnosis. Perhaps a cure will be found. Until that day comes, you must take a holistic approach to treatment. So start today, you really can make yourself better!

For those of you who are going through a hard time, the IBS network can provide great support and advice. The society is run for IBS sufferers, by IBS sufferers, and gives all kinds of helpful advice. There is a newsletter called 'Gut Reaction' which is produced four times a year. Local self-help groups exist in most areas. You'll find them listed in the useful addresses section at the back of the book.

TREATMENT PLAN FOR IBS

Symptoms

Constipation
Diarrhoea
Pain
Wind and distension

↓

Causes

Food intolerance
Infection
No obvious cause
Stress

↓

Treatment of cause

High-fibre diet   Stress management   Personality changes

Anti-stress plan
Relaxation
Self-hypnosis

↓

Treatment of symptoms

Pain	Constipation	Diarrhoea	Wind
Analgesics	High-fibre diet	Anti-diarrhoeals	Herbalism
Antispasmodics	Herbalism	High-fibre diet	Homoeopathy
Exercise	Homoeopathy	Herbalism	
Herbalism		Homoeopathy	
Homoeopathy			
Acupuncture			

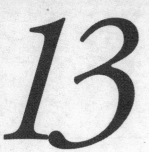

chapter thirteen

DIVERTICULITIS

D iverticula are small pouches that develop in the wall of the large bowel. In the West, they are found in approximately forty per cent of those over the age of sixty. However, they are very rare in the developing world, where the diet is higher in fibre and food is not subject to refining processes. The exact reason for their formation is not fully understood but, because of their association with increasing age, degenerative processes are probably involved. Undoubtedly, constipation is an important factor, where greatly increased pressure is required to force small quantities of hard, dry stool through the bowel. This rise in pressure can cause pouches to form at weak points in the wall of the descending colon. Diverticula in themselves do not cause symptoms but, if waste matter becomes trapped in them, they can become infected and inflamed producing a condition called diverticulitis.

Symptoms of diverticulitis

In some people, diverticulitis may show itself slowly, with a low-grade, nagging, left-sided abdominal pain and alternating constipation and diarrhoea. In others, the pain may be more intense, suddenly worsening, with constipation or diarrhoea. In a few cases, it may even be life-threatening, where the first sign is a massive rectal haemorrhage, which requires immediate transfusion in hospital. There is also a slight danger

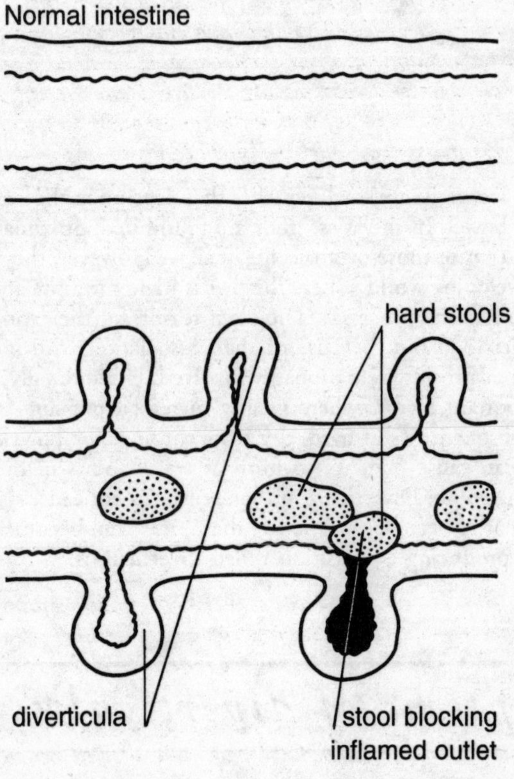

Normal intestine

hard stools

diverticula

stool blocking
inflamed outlet

Figure 13.1   Diverticula with hard stools

that one of the diverticula might perforate the bowel wall allowing its contents to leak into the abdominal cavity. This can either form a localised abscess or eventually lead to generalised peritonitis which is very dangerous, requiring an urgent operation.

Hilary is a fifty seven year old woman who had recently retired after twenty seven years as a librarian. She had looked forward to spending more time at home and having a generally less busy life. Three weeks after finishing work, her husband rang one morning and told me his wife was complaining of severe stomach pain. This had come on slowly over a few days and was mainly located down the left side of her abdomen. Hilary had suffered with constipation for some time but blamed this on her diet, which she intended to improve now that she had retired. The pain had suddenly become more severe through the night and she had started to be sick. On that particular morning, she had experienced some diarrhoea and had noticed her stools were streaked with blood.

On examination, she looked unwell and had a low-grade temperature of 38.9°C. Her abdomen was swollen and extremely tender on the left side. I explained to Hilary that pain of this degree, on the left side of the abdomen, which is associated with a period of constipation, is almost always from diverticulitis.

I considered sending Hilary to hospital but, as she was very upset at the idea, I decided to treat her at home, watching her very carefully for any signs of deterioration in her condition.

Initial treatment in the acute stages is with antibiotics and painkillers both given in large doses to try and prevent any complications of the diverticulitis. In fact, as there was a risk of Hilary vomiting back the medicine, I gave her an injection of morphine and benzyl-penicillin. I instructed her husband, Jeff, to call me immediately if the pain suddenly worsened.

I returned after evening surgery and Hilary looked a little brighter. The morphine had deadened the pain and allowed her to sleep. On examination, her temperature had come down by half a degree, her pulse rate had fallen and her stomach was less tender. I therefore felt it safe to leave her at home for the night, but called in the morning on my way to the surgery. She had had a rough night with pain and hot sweats, but she had finally managed some sleep and now felt much better.

Treatment continued over the following ten days with antibiotics and painkillers by mouth, but it was a full two weeks before Hilary felt well enough to be up and about. At that time, she still had some cramp-like pain in her stomach but I was able to relieve this with anti-spasmodic tablets.

Three months later, Hilary came back to see me, saying she was still suffering some discomfort in the lower stomach. She had intermittent attacks of nausea and also found that certain foods caused diarrhoea or constipation. It was certainly not allowing her to have the peaceful retirement she had dreamed about for so long.

Unfortunately, it is unusual to have a single attack of diverticulitis and then have no further problems. An after-effect of infection is the thickening of bowel wall, affecting the function of the muscles which push the faeces along the intestines. Usually the muscles become underactive, resulting in constipation, but occasionally they become twitchy, leading to diarrhoea and cramp-like pains.

Investigations

BARIUM ENEMA

The most valuable investigation is a special X-ray called a barium enema. Although it is not the most pleasant of tests, it is simple to carry out and reveals a great deal about the patient's condition. A small quantity of radio-opaque barium sulphate is passed into the rectum via a narrow tube and, by tilting the patient into the head-down position, the barium runs into the large intestine. It then fills any diverticula that are present, and these show up white on X-rays. This procedure only takes about thirty minutes and it is perfectly possible to go home again within an hour.

A common appearance is just a few pouches in the lowermost bowel, which generally give the patient little trouble in the future. With extensive diverticula, however, the chances of further problems are very high.

I needed to assess the severity of Hilary's condition, so I sent her to the hospital for a barium enema. Unfortunately the X-ray showed multiple diverticula extending well into her large intestine. I gently explained to Hilary that this was the reason for her continuing pain and disturbance of bowel habit. She was also running the risk of complications, including another infective episode similar to the one she had experienced or occasional and severe bleeding, intestinal obstruction or perforation.

Conventional treatment

Orthodox treatment is usually aimed at controlling the symptoms. If pain is the dominant feature, then analgesics, usually paracetamol, are prescribed. If constipation occurs, then a bulking laxative, such as Fybogel, is taken. Cramp-like pains are treated with an antispasmodic tablet and infection, with antibiotics. If the symptoms become too severe, admission to hospital is sometimes necessary (mainly to allow fluids to be given intravenously through a drip). Surgery is reserved for major complications, where the diseased segment of bowel is excised out.

While many people are quite happy to take a purely symptomatic approach, it does have the great drawback of not preventing recurrences, which are almost inevitable.

Alternative therapies

NATUROPATHY

While hospital admission may be life-saving if major complications arise, these can usually be avoided if the correct preventive care is taken. This is where natural therapy can be of great benefit.

High-fibre diet
A major cause of diverticulitis is constipation, where straining to pass hard, dry stools increases the pressure on the bowel wall, leading to the formation of the pouch-shaped diverticula. Constipation can usually be avoided with a high-fibre diet. Very few people will not become constipated on a diet which is low in fibre, but when I tell patients to increase the fibre in their diets, they become downcast at the thought

of having to sprinkle bran on all their food. Although bran is a very useful source of fibre, there are many other natural ways of taking it. About 25 to 30 grams of fibre are required each day to produce a soft, non-constipated stool. A reasonable quantity (at least five portions per day) of fruit, vegetables, nuts and pulses will provide the necessary amount of fibre.

Low-residue diet

In the acute phase of diverticulitis, the bowel lining is inflamed and infected, leading to pain, nausea and often diarrhoea. At this stage, fibre should be avoided as the bowel needs to rest. While a fluid only diet is acceptable for a couple of days, it may well take two to three weeks for the acute episode to settle. A low-residue diet is valuable at this time, as it still enables you to eat solids which have a minimum effect on the inflamed bowel. Your aim should be to eat as normally as possible, but avoiding all fruits, most vegetables, nuts, any wholegrain cereals or those containing bran wherever possible.

Breakfast

- Cereals including Rice Krispies, Special K or oatmeal porridge;
- Strained fruit juice;
- Egg, bacon or fish – not fried;
- White bread or toast;
- Butter, jelly, jam, honey or jelly marmalade;
- Tea or coffee.

Lunch and dinner

- Clear soup;
- Meat, fish, egg or cheese dish;
- Potatoes (preferably mashed), rice or spaghetti, marrow;
- White rolls;
- Pudding may include jelly, plain yoghurt, cake or biscuits.

HOMOEOPATHY

This method of treating illness is increasing in popularity, partly because it considers the patient as a whole being, but also because homoeopathic remedies are free of side-effects. As ever, the choice of remedy depends on personality as well as the nature of the abdominal symptoms.

- For individuals who are lively, cheerful, prefer warmth, do not like loud noise and experience sudden, griping pain, **Belladonna** 30c is the remedy of choice. It should be taken every hour, when the symptoms are severe and twice daily, as a preventative measure.
- **Bryonia** is for the quieter person who is rather shy. They often describe the pain as being like a stitch on the left side, with their abdomen feeling as if it is about to burst. Pressure makes the pain worse and it can be severe enough to prevent movement, thought or speech. Bryonia should be taken in the 6c potency.
- Violent, cutting, twisting pain just below the navel, relieved by passing wind or bending forwards, is suitable for the remedy **Colocynth**. It best suits the person who is irritable and domineering.
- **Magnesia phos** is excellent for the stoic type, where the pain is so violent that the patient cries out. This type of pain may be relieved by warmth, friction and pressure on the abdomen.

HERBAL THERAPY

‘ If any man can name all the properties of mint, he must know how many fish swim in the ocean. ’

Wilafried of Strabo (Twelfth Century)

I have prescribed peppermint tea many times since it eased my own stomach problem a decade ago. It is an antispasmodic and a digestive tonic, which is equally effective on the stomach or the bowel. The peppermint herb is widely used because it is so soothing. There are thought to be about thirty species of mint. Until the seventeenth century, all mints were used in much the same way. Today, peppermint is preferred in the West for medicinal purposes, whereas the Chinese use the field mint known as *bo he*. Garden mint (usually spearmint) is often used for children, as it is not as strong as peppermint.

An infusion of peppermint is made in much the same way as ordinary tea. The water, however, should be kept just off the boil, since the steam of vigorously boiling water disperses valuable, volatile oils. It must be made fresh each day and the quantity is sufficient for three cupfuls. Put 15 gm of dried peppermint (or 30 gm of the fresh herb) into a pot with a close fitting lid. Pour 500 mls of near-boiling water into the pot over the herb. Leave the mixture to infuse for ten minutes and then strain into a tea cup through a nylon sieve. You can store whatever is left in a jug in a cool place. Peppermint tea can be drunk hot or cold but is so much more soothing when taken hot.

Chamomile tea is a suitable alternative but the taste isn't as pleasant. It is made in exactly the same way. Slippery elm gruel, taken twice daily, reduces the inflammation of the bowel but, as many people find it tastes horrible, I rarely recommended it.

ACUPUNCTURE AND ACUPRESSURE

As dietary, homoeopathic and herbal remedies are effective and simple to use, I reserve acupuncture mainly for patients with resistant pain. Needles are placed into three specific points: Spleen 6, Stomach 29 and Ren 4. The needles are stimulated for twenty minutes. Often, total relief is felt, as soon as the stimulation begins. The treatment sessions are repeated twice a week for a month.

Acupressure over the points using the finger tips can also bring relief, but not as rapidly as the use of needles. The same points as those listed for acupuncture should be gently massaged for five minutes, three times a day.

HYPNOSIS

Diverticulitis often occurs at times of high stress. It is logical, therefore, to take measures to prevent stress levels becoming too high. For more on this subject, see the anti-stress plan (pages 139–141). Hypnosis is an excellent way of achieving deep relaxation. The therapist can also teach self-hypnosis, which can be used at any time. Psychological factors often contribute to pain – self-hypnosis can reduce tension and also relax the spasm in the intestinal muscles. The technique of putting yourself in a hypnotic trance is described fully in Chapter 3 and I would recommend it for everyone who suffers with diverticulitis.

Hilary preferred an alternative approach to managing her condition. However, she had not been following a healthy, high-fibre diet. In fact, she rarely ate breakfast and lunch consisted of a couple of sandwiches, made with white bread. Having spent a busy day at the library, Hilary would usually stop at the supermarket and buy a microwaveable, convenience meal for her supper. Not a grain of fibre in sight!

I advised Hilary to increase the amount of fibre she was eating. She also found that peppermint tea and Belladonna helped to control her

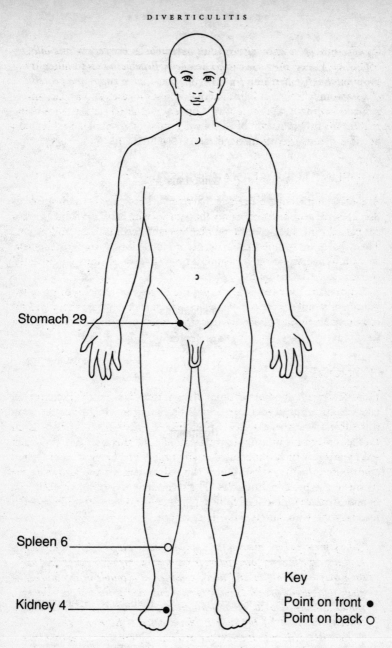

Stomach 29

Spleen 6

Kidney 4

Key

Point on front ●
Point on back ○

Figure 13.2   Acupuncture points for diverticulitis

symptoms. These days, diverticulitis only troubles her very occasionally. During attacks, she increases her intake of Belladonna and switches to the low-residue diet, for a few days. She now leads a happy and peaceful retirement.

TREATMENT PLAN FOR DIVERTICULITIS

Symptoms

Diarrhoea or constipation
Distension of abdomen
Nausea
Stools streaked with blood (in some cases)

Investigations

Case history
Rectal examination
Sigmoidoscopy

Treatment

Self-help

High-fibre diet
Exercise

Conventional medicines	Homoeopathy	Herbalism	Acupuncture
Antidepressants	Belladonna	Chamomile	Kidney 4
Antispasmodics	Bryonia	Peppermint	Spleen 6
Bulk laxatives	Colocynth	Slippery elm	Stomach 29
	Magnesium phosphate		

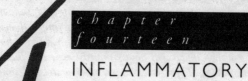

INFLAMMATORY BOWEL DISEASE

The appearance of blood in faeces can quite understandably be alarming for the sufferer. It is a sign of inflammation of the lining of the intestine, which has become friable and so bleeds. Infection and piles are the two most common causes, both of which are easily treatable and of short duration. Occasionally, however, a chronic inflammation develops, such as ulcerative colitis or Crohn's disease. The main symptom of both these conditions is bloody diarrhoea. These, together with colitis as a result of acute infections, are grouped under the term 'inflammatory bowel disease'.

Ulcerative colitis

Its very title virtually describes the disease process. Colitis is an inflammation of the colon which causes diarrhoea, usually with blood and mucus. In ulcerative colitis, the lining of the bowel becomes inflamed, eventually forming numerous, small ulcers, which bleed easily and profusely. The cause is unknown, but it is thought that an abnormality in the body's immune system might be a contributive factor. Initially, the disease only affects the rectum, but the rest of the large intestine can gradually become affected.

Martin is a twenty eight year old assistant in a local solicitor's. Approximately two years ago, he developed a sudden and violent episode of diarrhoea. He thought this was simply due to an infection and treated himself with rest, fluids and Imodium tablets. The attack lasted a week, which was longer than he expected, but he did not seek medical advice. Three weeks later, after a stressful time at work, the diarrhoea recurred. He thought that it was a reaction produced by tension, especially as it seemed to settle over the weekend. Once he returned to work, he noticed streaks of blood in his stools the following evening and, by morning, the bleeding had increased. By now, he was passing significant quantities of fresh blood and mucus, quite separately from any faeces. Although his stomach was uncomfortable, he did not experience a great deal of pain and had called me out because he was worried about the amount of blood he was losing.

On examination, there were few abnormalities. Although he didn't look well, the bleeding was not sufficient to cause anaemia. I was concerned, however, by the recurrent nature of the diarrhoea and the appearance of heavy bleeding, which suggested that Martin had developed ulcerative colitis.

INVESTIGATIONS

The diagnosis of ulcerative colitis can be confirmed by protoscopy. A proctoscope (a viewing instrument similar to a speculum) is gently inserted through the anus, permitting the doctor to look directly at the rectum. The patient can later be referred to hospital for a sigmoido-scopy which enables the specialist to see much further up the bowel.

MANAGEMENT

Ulcerative colitis can be a serious condition. While most attacks can be treated at home, some cases can be very severe with heavy bleeding and toxicity. This can then lead to circulatory collapse which needs hospital treatment with intravenous fluids.

Management is divided into two phases: dealing with the acute episode, followed by long-term prevention.

DEALING WITH THE ACUTE EPISODE

If the disease is confined to the rectum, the proctitis (inflammation of the rectum) is brought under control with local steroid preparations such as

Prednisolone suppositories, which are very simple to use. Enemas may also be of help (Predsol and Colifoam are the two most widely used). Sulphasalazine tablets (1 gm twice daily) may also be taken over a period of several months to prevent a relapse.

Where the disease is too far up the bowel to be reached with enemas, steroids are taken by mouth: Prednisolone in a dose of 60 mg daily and 1 gm of Sulphasalazine, twice daily.

Effectiveness of treatment is judged by a reduction in stool frequency and the disappearance of mucus and blood from the faeces. Once remission has been achieved, the dose of steroids is gradually reduced and stopped after a period of six to eight weeks. Sulphasalazine is best taken for at least three months. Some specialists may, however, continue it indefinitely as they feel it reduces the incidence of further attacks.

As each attack of ulcerative colitis is potentially dangerous, it must be treated vigorously and I have no hesitation in prescribing steroids immediately because they can be life-saving.

On examination, the lining of Martin's rectum looked very red and multiple ulcers were clearly visible. He was later given a sigmoidoscopy, which fortunately indicated the rest of his bowel was clear. I prescribed Prednisolone suppositories and Sulphasalazine tablets, which greatly improved his symptoms. He also found enemas helpful. The bleeding soon stopped and he was able to return to work after only a day's absence.

Doreen *was not as fortunate as Martin, as the ulcerative colitis extended well up into her large bowel. Her symptoms started ten years ago when, like Martin, she was in her twenties. Initially, the attacks came every couple of months but, having taken preventive measures, she had not suffered any problems for nearly two years. Unfortunately, she had recently lost her job and this, coupled with her mother's recent illness, meant that Doreen had been through a very stressful time. This had undoubtedly triggered off another episode of ulcerative colitis with diarrhoea, mucus and blood loss. I prescribed Prednisolone and Sulphasalazine, to which she reacted well but, as a considerable area of the bowel was affected, it took a month for her diarrhoea to settle completely.*

LONG-TERM MANAGEMENT

Alternative methods like herbalism and homoeopathy, which are slower to act are best reserved for long-term management.

Homoeopathy
The homeopathic remedies available for ulcerative colitis are:

- **Phosphorus 6c** where there is profuse bleeding and any pain or discomfort which is relieved by opening the bowels. The Phosphorus person is intelligent, bright and sensitive; usually tall and thin; feels better for eating. A warm environment suits such people but they do not like the dark.
- **Mercurius corr. 6c** is prescribed when the stools are hot and offensive-smelling and when passing them causes cutting pains. The discomfort persists for sometime afterwards.
- **Arsenicum 6c** is the remedy prescribed for the person who is typically chilly, restless and anxious, and who experiences burning pain in the abdomen, accompanied by vomiting. These symptoms worsen after midnight and are partly relieved by sipping hot drinks.

Herbal remedies

- Slippery elm, taken twice daily, will soothe the irritated intestinal lining.
- Try alternating this with astringent teas such as agrimony, taken three or four times daily.
- Include fresh chickweed in salads or take it as a warm infusion for its soothing and healing properties.

Boosting the immune system
The main key to this, is to keep the immune system (the body's natural defence mechanism), in as tip top condition as possible. This can be achieved through:

- **Control of Stress** This is certainly the most important step in the long-term control of ulcerative colitis. Time and again, I see patients who have no problems when life is going smoothly but, as soon as an upset occurs, their colitis symptoms flare up again.

  Some stressful situations are unavoidable, so it is vital to find some method of controlling them so they do not affect your health. Some patients use relaxation tapes or go to yoga classes. My own preference is self-hypnosis, as it is easy to learn and can be practised at virtually any time. Turn to the anti-stress plan (pages 139–141) for more ideas.

- **Exercise** All the systems of the body benefit from exercise, none more than the immune system. The exertion does not have to be too strenuous: a twenty minute walk each day, a swim at the local pool or a workout at the gym a couple of times a week. Exercising regularly takes some commitment, but it is vital to maintain your natural defences.
- **Diet** Processed, refined foods have a disastrous effect on the immune system. Switching to wholefoods, eating plenty of fresh fruit and vegetables will do much to improve the condition. As a high intake of fibre is needed, some of the vegetables should be eaten raw. Wheat may irritate the bowel, but other grains, such as brown rice and millet, are beneficial.
- **Vitamins** A high-potency multivitamin preparation should be taken, together with vitamin C (100 mg daily), and vitamin B6 (25 mg daily). It is most important to take vitamin B6 when on steroids.

For the long-term management of **Martin***'s condition, I suggested he take Phosphorus, as his symptoms and personality suited this homoeopathic remedy almost exactly. As his attack had followed a period of acute stress, I encouraged him to take up some activity which would help cope with it. He took up cycling in the hills, several times a week, as being outdoors helps him to concentrate on other things and forget his worries. He also paid more attention to his diet, avoided convenience foods and adopted a wholefood diet.*

*   **Doreen***, on the other hand, was best suited to Mercurius corr. In addition to this homoeopathic remedy, she also practises self-hypnosis to free her mind from worry and tension. Happily, she has had no problems since.*

Crohn's disease

This is the other main condition where the lining of the intestine becomes inflamed and swollen. In contrast to ulcerative colitis (where ulcers are the dominant feature), the parts of the gut which are affected generally appear very smooth, with only a few scattered ulcers. The cause of Crohn's disease is unknown but, again, it seems to be triggered off by

Normal intestine

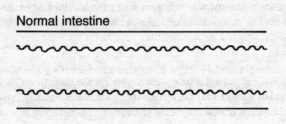

Ulcerative colitis

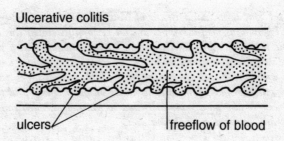

ulcers   freeflow of blood

Crohn's disease

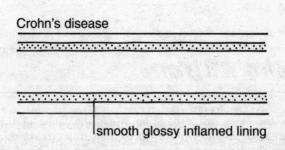

smooth glossy inflamed lining

Figure 14.1   Intestine showing Crohn's disease and ulcerative colitis

166

severe stress. There is also often a history of gastro-enteritis. Both stress and infection impair the immune system, so it is quite likely that Crohn's disease is the result of a disorder in the immune system. Unlike ulcerative colitis, the disease may involve any part of the alimentary tract, from the mouth to the anus, although the small intestine is usually the most commonly affected area. This may give rise to malabsorption of certain foodstuffs.

The predominant features of Crohn's disease are pain, diarrhoea and general malaise. Blood is often absent unless the large bowel is affected. A great deal of weight may be lost through malabsorption. If untreated, the disease can progress to the rest of the intestine producing abscesses, ulcers and skin tags, particularly around the anus.

INVESTIGATIONS

Sigmoidoscopy permits the rectum and the lower colon to be viewed directly, using an endoscope. As the rectum often looks normal on proctoscopy (see page 162), this investigation is essential. Most specialists will also carry out a colonoscopy (inspection of the colon with a viewing instrument).

MANAGEMENT OF ACUTE EPISODES

Each attack can cause severe damage to the intestine, so treatment with steroids is essential. The regime is similar to that used in ulcerative colitis but the response is slower. Pain is usually severe and if it is not relieved by steroids rapidly, then analgesics should be taken.

LONG-TERM MANAGEMENT

Crohn's disease is a chronic, relapsing condition. The aim in long-term care is to lead a normal life and keep attacks down to a minimum. Preventative measures include:

- Keeping the immune system in perfect working condition as described for ulcerative colitis earlier in this chapter (see pages 164–165). However, even more attention must be paid to the type of food eaten. It is necessary to have an extremely balanced diet, which provides a high level of unrefined carbohydrate and protein, from sources other than red meat (such as fish and chicken).

While some doctors are still reluctant to accept the role of diet in Crohn's disease, most now accept that food plays a major part. Naturopaths have treated this condition for some time by using an exclusion diet. The foodstuffs most likely to cause problems are wheat, corn, oats, dairy produce, red meats, citrus fruits, onions, coffee, tea, nuts, chocolate, food preservatives and yeast. Sufferers of Crohn's disease who have experimented with excluding these foods from their diets, have found it very successful;

- The homoeopathic remedies are as for ulcerative colitis (Phosphorus, Arsenicum and Mercurius corr.). These can be of benefit to all sufferers of the disease but, as treatment needs to be specific, it is advisable to consult a registered homoeopath;
- Acupuncture can produce dramatic results. The aim is to remove excesses of activity in the various pathways particularly the Stomach channel (see Figure 14.2). Pressure on the point midway between the navel and the breast bone will help when the symptoms are acute.

Mandy was only sixteen when she first experienced the symptoms of Crohn's disease. She had been on a school trip where the whole class was taken ill with food poisoning, after eating some infected chicken. All the other children had recovered quickly, but Mandy's diarrhoea persisted and she had developed attacks of cramp-like, right-sided abdominal pain. Mandy was at a difficult age, and didn't take much notice of medical advice. Consequently, she suffered badly in the first few years. Now she is in her late twenties and is far more sensible. Initially, I prescribed steroids to clear her acute symptoms. It was in fact several months before I could wean her off them completely. I advised her to follow the preventative measures (listed above) to help with the long-term management of the condition. Her symptoms have now stabilised and thankfully, she has not experienced any complications.

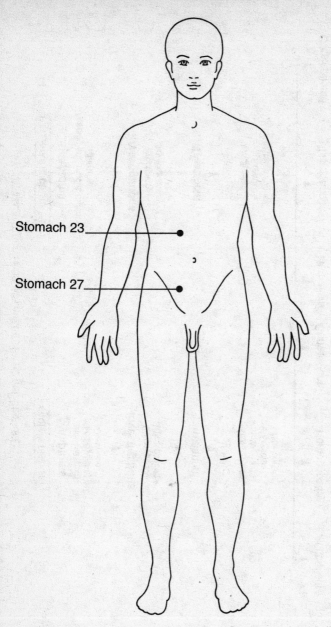

Stomach 23

Stomach 27

Figure 14.2   Acupuncture points for inflammatory bowel disease

TREATMENT PLAN FOR INFLAMMATORY BOWEL DISEASE

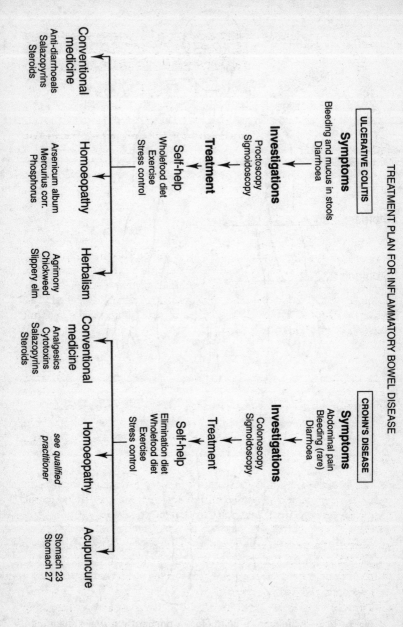

ULCERATIVE COLITIS

Symptoms
Bleeding and mucus in stools
Diarrhoea

Investigations
Proctoscopy
Sigmoidoscopy

Treatment

Self-help
Wholefood diet
Exercise
Stress control

Conventional medicine
Anti-diarrhoeals
Salazopyrins
Steroids

Homoeopathy
Arsenicum album
Mercurius corr.
Phosphorus

Herbalism
Agrimony
Chickweed
Slippery elm

CROHN'S DISEASE

Symptoms
Abdominal pain
Bleeding (rare)
Diarrhoea

Investigations
Colonoscopy
Sigmoidoscopy

Treatment

Self-help
Elimination diet
Wholefood diet
Exercise
Stress control

Conventional medicine
Analgesics
Cytotoxins
Salazopyrins
Steroids

Homoeopathy
see qualified practitioner

Acupuncure
Stomach 23
Stomach 27

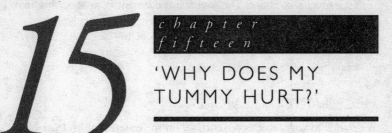

chapter fifteen

'WHY DOES MY TUMMY HURT?'

A cute abdominal pain is the most common reason for emergency hospital admissions. Many of these turn out to be unnecessary. This chapter is designed as a guide to help you achieve a likely diagnosis and to decide whether any immediate action is needed. The treatment for the different conditions is dealt with in the relevant chapters of this book.

Manifestations of abdominal pain

Pain in the abdomen may manifest itself in many ways. Each variation in pain, however, is slightly different and this may help to point to the diagnosis. A few general principles to bear in mind are:

- **Onset** The onset of pain is sudden when an organ is perforated, for example a stomach ulcer, but builds up gradually in other conditions, such as appendicitis, gall stones, diverticulitis, urinary infections and gastro-enteritis;
- **Type** Pain from the intestine is colicky (it comes and goes, making the sufferer move about). Pain from a perforation, or an inflamed

appendix, is constant. The slightest movement is so agonising that the patient finds relief in lying completely still;

- **Site** The typical sites of pain are shown below (see Figure 15.1). As there is often a degree of overlap, this diagram is not a guarantee of the diagnosis, but intended to be helpful pointer.

MISCELLANEOUS FEATURES

A detailed history which concentrates on the onset, type and site of the pain should be coupled with any other significant features to provide an accurate diagnosis. These include:

- Persistent indigestion suggests the possibility of an ulcer (see pages 35–51);
- Bleeding from the rectum points to diverticulitis (see pages 151–160), ulcerative colitis (pages 161–165), Crohn's disease (pages 165–169) or, in rare cases, cancer (pages 176–184);
- Profuse diarrhoea is likely to indicate gastro-enteritis (see page 53);
- Progressive constipation may precede intestinal obstruction (see pages 93–95), diverticulitis (pages 151–160) or irritable bowel syndrome (pages 123–150);
- Drugs may cause severe abdominal pain, for example those used for arthritis;
- Age is an important factor: appendicitis tends to occur in the young, gall stones and ulcers often present themselves around forty, whereas diverticulitis is most common in the elderly;
- In simple inflammation, pressure causes extreme tenderness. In some cases, such as a perforation or appendicitis, pain increases when the hand is taken away (rebound tenderness). It may also indicate peritonitis, which necessitates an operation.

Case studies

The following six cases illustrate different forms of abdominal pain to which the principles listed above can be applied.

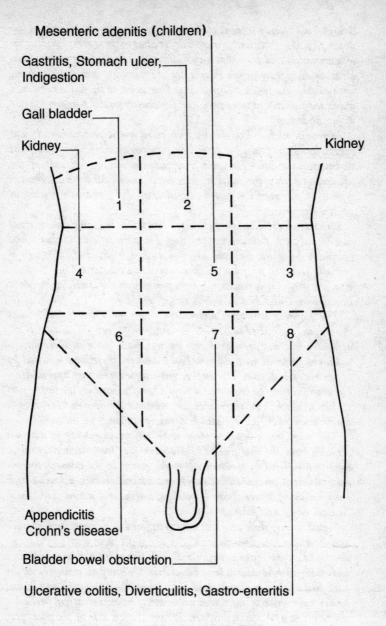

Figure 15.1   Sites of abdominal pain

Bridget is a twenty three year old secretary, who developed pain in the upper part of her stomach one evening. It came on in waves, building up to a crescendo and then slowly subsiding. In between spasms, the pain virtually disappeared. Two hours later, she started to vomit and suffered with profuse diarrhoea. When I visited her at home the following day, I found she was still in some pain and felt acutely tender over the left side of her abdomen.

Her pain had a slow onset which ruled out a perforation. It was colicky in nature (pain free periods in between attacks), which is typical of intestinal spasm. The pain was situated on the left side of the abdomen which is the position of the lower bowel. All these features are typical of an infective gastro-enteritis and her condition settled in twenty-four hours.

Deidre, of a similar age to Bridget, had much the same experience of abdominal pain, followed by vomiting. The pain differed in that it had gradually built up over the previous twelve hours and, although it initially occurred in spasms, had now become constant. On examination, she was acutely sensitive to light pressure on the lower, right side of her abdomen and had a slightly raised temperature.

The diagnosis was acute appendicitis (see page 55) and Deidre was immediately admitted to hospital for emergency surgery. Fortunately the appendix had not perforated and she was back home in three days.

David, a seven year old boy, had a cold for three days followed by upper abdominal pain. His mother was worried about an appendicitis. On examination, he cried out in pain when I pressed on the upper part of his stomach but there was no rebound tenderness. He had a temperature of 39°C. He also had enlarged glands in his neck.

The pain was constant rather than colicky suggesting it was not actually from the intestine. The diagnosis was mesenteric adenitis, a condition suffered by children where the glands in the stomach become enlarged. It is preceded by a cough or cold and there is always a high temperature. The condition is viral in origin and settled with paracetamol syrup and bedrest.

Geoff is sixty three and had always suffered with a sensitive stomach and irregular bowel movements. On the golf course that morning, he developed a cramp-like pain down the left side of his abdomen. He then had severe diarrhoea with some blood in it. Opening his bowels eased the pain but, by the time I examined him, it had built up again and he was tender over most of his lower abdomen. On examination he had a temperature and was acutely tender over the left side of the abdomen, but there was no rebound effect.

The onset was gradual which ruled out a perforation. His pain was colicky in nature suggesting it came from the intestine. At the age of sixty three, the most likely diagnosis for pain and bloody diarrhoea is acute diverticulitis. As he had passed some blood, it was imperative to rule out bowel cancer, although this was unlikely as pain is not usually a feature of cancerous growths. I thus referred him to the hospital for an internal examination and happily it was clear. The initial pain he experienced soon settled down with fluids and antibiotics. (For more information of diverticulitis, see Chapter 13.)

Brenda, *a forty year old woman, had long history of indigestion which she treated herself using various remedies she had bought from the chemist. One morning the burning sort of pain she usually experienced suddenly changed to absolute agony. On examination, her abdomen was absolutely rigid, and extremely tender to the touch. The pain was located in the upper central part of the abdomen and there was positive rebound tenderness. The slightest movement made her cry out.*

The sudden, severe onset of pain suggested a perforation. In fact, Brenda's was a classic case of a perforated stomach ulcer (see pages 35–51). When this happens, acid from the stomach can leak into the abdominal cavity, causing peritonitis. Fortunately, this is rare, as early drug treatment of ulcers is so effective these days. Once perforation has occurred, the only treatment is an operation to sew up the hole in the stomach wall. Brenda was in hospital for ten days and made a full recovery.

Alison *is a thirty eight year old secretary who had severe, right-sided, upper abdominal pain, which was making her roll around in agony. The pain came and went every three minutes and she was vomiting increasingly frequently. It had been present for several hours, but had suddenly become much worse. She had suffered milder episodes of pain over the previous year and experienced an intolerance of fatty food.*

The onset of pain was gradual, but suddenly became much more severe suggesting an obstruction or possibly a perforation. It was colicky in nature, which also indicated an obstruction. These symptoms were typical of gall stones (see pages 80–90) and the sudden increase in pain indicated that a stone had become stuck in the outlet of the gall bladder. Treatment with analgesics and muscle relaxants allowed the stone to fall back and the obstruction to clear.

From these cases, you can see how doctors approach the diagnosis of abdominal pain and I hope it will give you an idea of the diagnosis, if you ever suffer from any of these symptoms yourself.

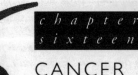

16

CANCER

E very day, as part of the continuous growth and repair process which takes place in the human body, some 500 billion new cells are formed. Occasionally, defective cells are produced, some of which may escape the policing activities of the immune system and begin to multiply extremely fast. Rapid, uncontrolled growth is characteristic of cancer cells. A rapidly-dividing colony of cancer cells becomes a tumour, which unfortunately can invade normal tissue. If cancer cells spread to other parts of the body via the blood or lymph glands, then secondary tumours may develop.

Overall, cancer affects more men than women and older people rather than youngsters. In Great Britain alone, 500,000 people develop digestive cancer commonly in the stomach and large intestine. The faster the tumour can be diagnosed, the greater the chance there is of a cure, as it can be removed completely before the cancer has a chance to spread. Once the cancer cells reach other parts of the body, then complete eradication becomes more difficult.

Warning signs

A single, simple test to detect cancer in the body has yet to be developed. Perhaps, one day it will be possible to have a sample of blood tested each year to check whether any cancer has developed. For now, we must rely on early warning signs. For digestive cancers these are:

- Persistent indigestion;
- A change in bowel habit, either constipation or diarrhoea, which is unrelated to alterations in diet;
- Any bleeding from the mouth or anus;
- Unexplained weight loss.

These are not infallible signs of cancer. Nine times out of ten, these symptoms have more innocent causes, but they must nevertheless not be ignored as early diagnosis is vital, in cancer. If you develop any of these symptoms, please go and see your GP immediately.

Causes

The most likely reason for cancer is damage to the immune system where it loses the ability to destroy the abnormal cells as soon as they are formed. This theory is supported by several factors:

- The start of cancer can often be dated back to a major stressful event, such as a bereavement, redundancy or divorce. Stress is known to suppress the immune system. Cancer is also more common in people who constantly worry, in those who do not attempt to manage their stress levels and those who bottle up their anger;
- Our natural defences become less efficient as we grow older. Cancer is in fact more common in the elderly;
- The immune system can be affected by external factors (carcinogens), all of which have been linked to cancer. These include: cigarette smoke, radiation and asbestos fibres. Pollution in its varying forms, has been shown to damage the immune system.

Prevention

Cancer prevention involves a healthy diet and lifestyle, coping with stress, avoiding carcinogens and a positive mental attitude.

- **Changes in diet** The immune system is boosted by a fresh wholefood diet containing plenty of fresh fruit and vegetables. This has the added benefit of preventing constipation, which has been linked to large bowel cancer. In those countries where people eat high-fibre diets, there is a much lower incidence of stomach and bowel cancers than in places where the food is subject to refining processes. This is especially true of Western countries and Britain is no exception. The supplement, beta carotene has been shown to be beneficial as it makes cancer cells more vulnerable to the body's immune system. This should be taken daily and should preferably be combined with vitamin E.
- **Healthy lifestyle** The feeling of well being when we are fully fit, influences all parts of the body including the immune system. Regular exercise combined with plenty of rest and relaxation will achieve this.
- **Avoiding carcinogens** Smokers are twenty five times more likely to develop digestive cancers, than non-smokers. Eighty per cent of stomach cancers occur in those who smoke. Although it is stating the obvious to say that all forms of cigarettes should be banned, very few people take heed.
- **Relief of stress** If you are a worrier, then it is vital to find a way to deal with this in a positive way. It is virtually impossible to do this on your own and I would advise everyone with this type of personality, or who has recently experienced a major stressful event, to seek help from a counsellor. (For more on this subject, turn to the anti-stress plan on pages 139–141.)

Screening for cancer of the digestive system

The value of screening programmes is indisputable. The cure for cancer of the cervix in women has soared since the introduction of regular smears for all women. However, as the short-term cost of screening for stomach and bowel cancer is high, it has yet to be offered as a matter of course. Whichever government is in power, it appears that they fail to consider that such a procedure could save millions of pounds in the future. Perhaps this is because they fear they will be voted out before the benefits of screening have outweighed the initial outlay. Nevertheless, many specialists are pressing for screening programmes for digestive cancers. It is estimated that an endoscopic examination of the stomach for everyone with chronic indigestion would detect seventy five per cent of stomach cancers before they have spread. An even higher figure is quoted for bowel cancer, where detection is much easier. Tumours in the large intestine bleed very early on, although blood loss may be so small that it is not visible to the naked eye. However, a simple dipstick test is available, which takes two minutes to perform and can be carried out in any GP's surgery. If everyone over forty had a sample of faeces tested each year then eighty per cent of all bowel cancers would be detected, early enough for there to be a chance of complete recovery.

It has also been shown that cancer in the bowel may develop from little polyps (wart-like growths). These can remain in a benign state for many years, before becoming cancerous. It may, therefore, be of benefit to examine everyone internally and remove all these polyps, before they have a chance to change. This view is supported by many cancer specialists.

Treatment

No branch of medicine can offer a certain cure for cancer. It is sensible to consider all forms of therapy, to listen to what specialists, qualified homoeopaths and other alternative medicine practitioners have to say. It is important to adopt the strategy which appeals to you and to avoid fanatics at all cost. Depending on the kind of cancer you have, and the stage it has reached, you may need to combine several forms of treatment.

Conventional Treatment

SURGERY

For most cancers, including those of the stomach and intestines, the main chance of a complete cure is through an operation which removes the tumour.

Irene is a fifty one year old woman who discovered blood in her faeces, one day. Tests revealed a tumour, half way up her large intestine. Irene dreaded the thought of an operation but she didn't have any choice. Her tumour was small and had been detected early so her chances of long-term survival were excellent. She was admitted to hospital the following week and the cancerous area was easily removed. She made a fast recovery and was discharged six days later. Hopefully, Irene will have no further problems.

RADIOTHERAPY AND CHEMOTHERAPY

Sometimes the tumour is either too large to remove completely or, by the time of operation, the cancer has already spread to other parts of the body. When this occurs, it may be possible to treat the cancer with radiation or with anticancer drugs. These treatments kill the cancer cells but unfortunately damage the body's normal cells. In addition, they suppress the immune system, reducing the body's natural ability to fight disease. It is therefore very important, when considering either radiation or chemotherapy, to discuss fully with your specialist how these ill-effects can be minimised.

Alternative treatment

As each cancer is different, it is often difficult to advise which form of treatment is needed. However, as the cause may well be related to a deficiency in the immune system (which is affected negatively by conventional treatment), complimentary medicine must also be taken to boost the body's natural defences.

The three simple rules to boost the immune system still apply:

- **Remove stress** Relaxation is important and more advanced methods may need to be learnt like meditation and self-hypnosis. The anti-stress plan (pages 139–141) may also give you a few ideas.
- **Eat a healthy diet** One of the main principles of a diet to fight cancer, is to detoxify the body and thereby mobilise its own healing powers. Such diets focus on raw food (unprocessed food with no additives or colourings), which should be eaten as fresh as

possible. This provides a high-nutrient, low-calorie diet, since it contains fresh vegetables, fruit, nuts and seeds. Its high-fibre content helps the detoxification process. Processed foods should be avoided, and nutritional supplements in the form of high doses of vitamin C and beta carotene are recommended.

- **Take regular exercise** As the immune system thrives on exercise, some form should be taken on most days. Even if you don't feel well, taking a short walk can be beneficial.

These three steps are excellent ways to start repairing the body's defences but, as cancer is a serious condition, other methods are needed as well.

HOMOEOPATHY

The homoeopathic view of cancer is that it represents a profound breakdown in health on all levels. The aim of treatment, therefore, is to completely rebuild the immune system. Home-prescribing is not really appropriate in such circumstances and it is vital to seek the help of an experienced homoeopath who will prescribe the specific remedies suited to your particular case and personality, as well as constitutional treatment.

It is my own view that anyone with cancer, or who has had cancer, should continue with homoeopathic therapy although this may often need to be combined with conventional treatment.

Positive Thinking

‹ *Tell me straight doctor, is there any hope for me at all?* ›

Positive thinking has been shown to have a tremendous stimulating effect on the immune system and on the healing of cancerous cells. A group of researchers in London recently found a seventy five per cent survival rate among cancer patients who showed a fighting spirit, compared to twenty two per cent who responded to their illness with feelings of hopelessness.

My whole approach to cancer changed ten years ago when Edith, a fifty six year old woman came to see me. Edith had ignored symptoms of persistent indigestion and increasing weight loss for many months. By the time she was investigated by a specialist, her stomach cancer was too advanced to be removed. The consultant told her there was no orthodox treatment available to heal the tumour. As every patient has a right to know the true facts relating to their case, I explained as gently as I could that nineteen out of twenty people will die in six months when cancer is discovered at such a late stage.

Instead of bursting into tears, Edith's eyes lit up. 'But what about the twentieth?' she shouted. 'What happens to them?'

I explained to her that, very occasionally, a patient survives, but that it was difficult to say why.

'Then I shall be that twentieth person,' stated Edith, with no trace of doubt in her voice.

By conceding that people sometimes recover, I had unknowingly given Edith something to fight for. Miraculously, this conversation happened over ten years ago and Edith is still alive and well today. Her case completely changed my approach to seemingly incurable illness. So now, if nine out of ten people with a certain disease are expected to die, instead of telling all ten they will probably succumb, I always stress they could very well be the one who survives. To achieve this, you have to change, to deal with the factors which may have contributed to the cancer.

Ted was sixty when he developed bowel cancer and the affected area was removed. The specialist was worried, however, that the cancerous cells had spread to the surrounding lymph glands which meant a recurrence was likely in the future. Ted immediately made the resolution that he was going to see his grandchildren grow up. His words revealed a fighting spirit but I told him that he would need more than determination to achieve his aim – he would need to change his personality, deep down.

He always had a tendency to become angry, both with himself and others. Ted had to change completely, learning to love himself, despite his shortcomings and to adopt a more tolerant attitude. I am convinced that unconditional love (both for yourself and others) is the most powerful stimulant to the immune system. Ted found help at his church. There, he developed his faith, learnt forgiveness, and experienced peace and love, all of which changed him totally. Since then, he has never lost his will to live, or his positive attitude. In himself, he is now a much happier person. The change occurred over two years ago and Ted is still alive and well today.

Conclusion

> IMPORTANT
> Cancer can be beaten, but only with the combined approach of
> orthodox treatment and the healing powers of your own body.
> Never ignore the advice of specialists, as initial treatment may
> produce an immediate cure.

In order to fight cancer, you must ask yourself these questions:

- Do you love yourself enough to take good care of your body and
  your mind?
- Do you eat moderately, avoiding too much sugar, caffeine and fat?
- Are there plenty of fresh fruit and vegetables in your diet?
- Do you avoid most processed, additive-laden foods?
- Do you exercise?
- Are you self-motivated?
- Do you seek activities that give you joy and satisfaction?
- Do you forgive easily?
- Do you love yourself and those around you?
- Do you feel the world is a beautiful place worth living in?

These factors are very important in determining our state of health and
our will to live. With a positive attitude, anything is possible.

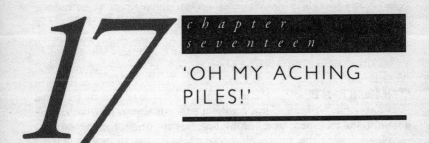

17

'OH MY ACHING PILES!'

> *'Doctor, I think I've got piles.'*
> *'Doctor, I'm in such pain from my piles.'*

S carcely a day goes by in the surgery without my hearing one of these comments. Considering they are so tiny, piles produce great suffering for so many with over fifty per cent of people in Great Britain experiencing them at some time in their lives.

What are piles and how are they formed?

Piles (haemorrhoids) are painful lumps that protrude from the anus. For many years, they were assumed to be a form of varicose vein. Recently, however, this theory has been discredited as untrue. Piles are in fact a protrusion of the lining of the bowel through the anus. This lining normally has a degree of flexibility to allow stretching as the stool passes through it. However, if the person is constipated, straining forces the lining downwards and it can then become trapped in the muscles of the anal sphincter (prolapse). This results in swelling and the increased

184

production of mucus which leaks on to the perineal skin, causing irritation and soreness. The inflamed lining also may bleed, usually in small amounts. However, significant blood loss may occasionally occur. Sometimes, the swelling within the anal canal may lead the patient to think that defaecation is incomplete, provoking further straining and therefore worsening the condition. If the lining becomes lax it will eventually stay outside the anus and the patient may find that manual replacement is needed. Occasionally, a strangulation occurs, where the blood supply to the trapped lining becomes impaired, causing extreme pain.

Young people are particularly prone to piles, as they have very strong anal muscles which cause additional trauma to the prolapsing lining. As gravity also plays a part, the popular habit of perusing newspapers and magazines on the toilet for prolonged periods of time, increases the downwards pressure.

Finally, even a normal excretory effort will, after many years, result in some degree of prolapse of the anal lining. Thus piles are often present in the elderly, although they may not experience any symptoms, as at this stage in life, the anus is invariably lax, allowing the piles to slide in and out without any discomfort.

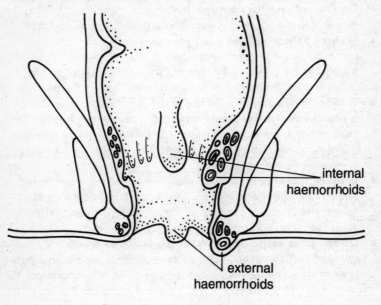

Figure 17.1   The formation of piles

In summary, haemorrhoids can be divided into three types:

- **Stage 1** where the piles are completely internal and patients complain of perineal irritation, incomplete defaecation and a constant desire to open the bowels. Bleeding may also occur;
- **Stage 2** where the piles prolapse out of the anus after defaecation;
- **Stage 3** where the haemorrhoids require manual replacement after defaecation.

Symptoms of piles

Many people do not like talking about their bowel habits and become embarrassed if asked to describe their symptoms. To overcome this, I use direct questions which only require a 'Yes' or 'No' answer.

- **Do you suffer with constipation?** As the major cause of piles is excessive straining there is inevitably a history of constipation.
- **Is there pain when you open your bowels?** Piles are often very sore especially if they prolapse. There is often an associated split in the anal lining, produced by the hard stool. This is called an anal fissure and can be the reason for a sudden increase in the pain.
- **Is there irritation around the anus?** The medical term for this is pruritus and usually occurs early in the development of haemorrhoids. Inadequate hygiene is the most common cause of pruritus, but it is also a major symptom of internal piles because of excess mucus production.
- **Is there bleeding from the anus?** The bright red blood from surface capillaries of an inflamed anal lining is characteristic of haemorrhoids. Blood loss may vary from a smearing on the toilet paper, to quite large amounts of fresh blood.
- **Do the piles come down?** While most people suffer some symptoms of piles as soon as they develop, in others the first sign is when they prolapse out of the anus. Initially, this may go unnoticed and the patient may complain of incomplete defaecation or a persistent desire to open the bowels.

Simon, *a thirty two year old computer operator, had felt some discomfort after opening his bowels and on examining himself found small, fleshy swellings. Although, this is the first time that many people realise they have piles, they are in fact quite advanced by this stage and will have been there for some months. He answered 'Yes' to all the questions listed above, so I was confident of the diagnosis of piles, simply from his answers.*

    Christine, *however, only complained of increasing rectal bleeding and was terrified she had cancer. She was a forty one year old manager of a local clothing business and had always enjoyed good health, apart from her bowels being rather stubborn. She first experienced constipation when she went to university (it is a common condition among students who tend to have a poor quality diet). A week previously she had noticed what she thought was blood on the toilet paper. Over the following few days, Christine's bleeding increased until there was no doubt in her mind that something very sinister was going on. She did not feel any anal irritation, pain or experience prolapse.*

BLEEDING FROM THE ANUS

Nearly all cases of rectal bleeding are due to piles. However, it is necessary to exclude the less common conditions which include:

- An anal fissure with bleeding from the split in the bowel lining;
- Inflammation of the bowel, usually from infection which makes the rectal lining very friable;
- Ulcerative colitis or diverticulitis (see Chapters 13 and 14);
- Simple rupture of a blood vessel from excessive straining;
- Very rarely, blood loss due to cancer.

Investigations

Examination of the anus and rectum is absolutely essential for anyone with rectal bleeding to exclude the possibility of a cancerous growth. These are uncommon but must not be missed, as the chances of recovery are high if the cancer is diagnosed at an early stage.

Everyone dreads the thought of an examination of the anal area. However, these examinations are a matter of routine for doctors who carry them out every day. This is also the reason why many doctors may seem insensitive to their patient's embarrassment.

- **Inspection** It is impossible to inspect your own anal area but often the diagnosis is obvious if the piles are visible.
- **Palpation** Digital examination is performed wearing a polythene glove, lubricated with K-Y jelly. If this is carried out gently and slowly, then discomfort is minimal. It is when doctors rush the procedure that anal spasms occur, resulting in pain. Examination enables any growths to be felt but, because internal piles are easily flattened, they cannot normally be felt with the palpating finger.
- **Proctoscopy** This is the most useful test for anyone with suspected internal piles. The proctoscope is made of stainless steel and is a very similar instrument to the speculum used for cervical smears. By passing the well-lubricated distal end gently through the anal opening, the lining can be viewed directly.
- **Sigmoidoscopy** If there is still any doubt as to the reason for the bleeding, it is necessary to carry out a further investigation, using a sigmoidoscope. This is a similar procedure to proctoscopy, but the sigmoidoscope is much longer and enables the whole of the rectum to be viewed. On occasions, diverticulitis, ulcerative colitis or rectal cancer can be discovered in this way. If piles are suspected, but are not found on proctoscopy, then no cause for the bleeding is ever found. In such cases, it must be assumed that a blood vessel has ruptured from straining too hard.

On examining Christine there were no external piles visible, simply some scratch marks as a result of itching in that area. On palpation, no abnormalities were discovered. Christine looked at me with absolute horror when I explained she would need a proctoscopy but patients are always surprised at how little discomfort it causes. By shining a light through the proctoscope I could visualise three internal piles, one of which was gently oozing blood from an inflamed artery. There was no sign of any cancer. She was mightily relieved to find the bleeding was due to piles, as she had convinced herself that cancer was the underlying cause. The examination had taken less than five minutes from start to finish and had been well worth the temporary discomfort, simply to set her mind at rest. In Simon's case, three soft fleshy swellings were protruding through the anus. The diagnosis was, therefore, confirmed to be piles although, as he had suffered some slight bleeding, it was necessary to check him internally. Simon's rectum appeared healthy. There was obviously no other cause for his bleeding other than prolapsed piles.

The best method of treatment for piles, whether orthodox or natural, is the subject of controversy. Many years of experience have shown me how successfully conventional and alternative medicine can work together.

Conventional treatment

STAGE 1

At this stage the piles are internal. The following regime is simple to implement and usually works in two to three days:

- As they are located inside the rectum, suppositories which contain an anti-inflammatory steroid and a local anaesthetic are effective. Anusol and Proctosedyl are the most popular.
- In the absence of any evidence of bacteriological infection, antibiotic creams should be avoided as the perineal skin is very delicate and sensitivity rashes are common.
- Any constipation should be cleared with a high-fibre intake and a bulking laxative, such as Fybogel.
- Prolonged straining and the reading of magazines while seated on the toilet should be stopped!

STAGE 2

At this stage, the piles protrude through the anal canal but easily slide back in. Initial treatment is as for stage 1; the condition will settle in the majority of cases. If not, the following are useful in persistent cases.

- An injection of five per cent phenol in vegetable oil. It is carried out in a hospital outpatient department, but only takes two to three minutes. It is very simple and rarely painful. The injection is given into the anal lining above the base of the pile causing the lining to shrink and draw the piles back into the anal canal. Further contraction over a few weeks means the piles eventually disappear.

- On the rare occasion where injections are ineffective, a surgical procedure is necessary. The most preferable is an anal stretch, which does not require any cutting. Maximum dilatation to six or eight fingerbreadths will stretch the anal muscles, enabling defaecation without excessive effort. Any prolapsed piles will not undergo any further strangulation and will reduce in size. The whole stretching procedure takes only a few minutes, but is done under anaesthetic as it can be very painful!

STAGE 3

Where the piles remain outside the anus permanently and can only be replaced manually, the treatment consists of:

- A high-fibre diet anti-inflammatory suppositories and bulk laxatives in the first instance;
- If this is unsuccessful, it may be necessary to have the piles surgically removed. By this stage, they are too big to respond to anal stretching and injections. Haemorrhoidectomy, as the surgical procedure is known, involves removing a section of the anal lining which is sufficient to prevent prolapse of the piles, but not enough to narrow the anus, through excessive scarring. This procedure is reserved for those patients who have tried every other method of treatment with little success.

In reality, I can only remember one case of anal stretching and one haemorrhoidectomy in my practice during the past ten years. Although some doctors believe in the removal of piles, my own feeling is that operations for any condition should be avoided if there is an effective alternative. The advantage of practising both conventional and natural medicine, is that I can use the benefits of both, often preventing the need for surgery. In the treatment of any of the three stages of piles, my initial approach is to use anti-inflammatory suppositories and to cure constipation. If the piles persist, I suggest complementary medicine.

Alternative therapies

SELF-HELP

- **Diet** Sensible eating habits, providing enough dietary fibre, will alleviate and in fact help to prevent piles by easing the pressure on the lower bowel. Approximately 25 gm of fibre should be eaten each day. This is not difficult to achieve by eating vegetables, fruit and pulses (see pages 155–156).
- **Exercise** Regular exercise improves the circulation in the area of the piles and also helps clear constipation. Any form is beneficial and only a few minutes each day is needed.
- **Hot and cold treatment** The use of a hot pack for five minutes followed by an ice pack for twenty minutes applied to the perineal area will help to shrink a painful pile.
- **Vitamin supplements** Piles respond, albeit slowly, to vitamin B6, 25 mg daily. If there is blood loss, it is advisable to take iron, folic acid and vitamin B12 to restore red blood cells.

Christine's piles were internal and she experienced intermittent bleeding and some anal irritation (stage 1). Her lifestyle was generally sedentary with most of her working day spent at a desk. This left her little time for exercise. Her diet consisted mainly of convenience food, usually low in fibre.

It is amazing how the simplest of changes in lifestyle can be beneficial to our health. By changing her fibre intake to 25 gm per day and taking a thirty minute walk every lunchtime, Christine quickly noticed that her bowel habits became more comfortable. A week's course of anti-inflammatory suppositories, inserted twice daily, completely stopped the bleeding and discomfort. Christine has remained well ever since, with no further trouble. Perhaps the threat of an operation helped her to carry out the necessary changes to her lifestyle!

Over ninety per cent of people with piles find their condition improves with suppositories, changes in diet and increased exercise. Occasionally, this regime does not work which can be for two reasons: either (as in Simon's case) the piles are already severe by the time treatment is sought or, more commonly, the person is not prepared to stick to the recommended changes. After the first couple of weeks, most people tend to slip back into the way they have lived for many years. Maintaining regular exercise, and a high-fibre diet is more difficult than it sounds. In these circumstances, I then turn to other methods of natural treatment.

HERBAL TREATMENT

These remedies are most effective for prolapsing piles:

- Pilewort (lesser celandine), which is available as an ointment, should be applied three times daily and after each bowel movement, to relieve pain, ease the inflammation and reduce the size of the piles;
- Distilled witch hazel may also be applied frequently, especially if the piles are very painful;
- An infusion of yarrow herb is useful for its astringency and its influence on blood vessels. It is taken cold in a dosage of 45–60 mls (three to four tablespoons), three times per day. It can also be applied as a compress.

HOMOEOPATHY

For people who do not like using conventional medication, then homoeopathic suppositories, instead of the conventional type, can be used. Hamamelis is available in this form but may have to be ordered through your local health food store. I only prescribe it in ointment form, which can be used both externally and internally.

In cases where the piles keep recurring, then homoeopathic remedies, which are taken by mouth, are of great value. This is one of the few situations where the choice of medication can be chosen quickly from the symptoms. While personality plays an important part in the choice of remedy, in piles, it would appear that a particular type of person experiences a particular type of symptom. The remedies I commonly prescribe include:

- **Hamamelis**, for bleeding and when there is a bruised feeling around the anus;
- **Nux vomica** where there is itching and constipation;
- **Aesculus** for backache and where there is dry itching and burning;

- **Aloes** when the piles look like a bunch of grapes and there is constipation with occasional episodes of explosive diarrhoea;
- **Pulsatilla** where there is continuous mucus production. This is particularly useful in pregnancy;
- **Hypericum** when the piles are very sensitive and bleed easily.

Simon, who really had quite severe prolapsing piles, was keen to try a natural approach. The homoeopathic remedy which best suited his problem was Aloes. He took these three times per day over a period of two months. Of the various creams, he preferred the pilewort as this was the most soothing and seemed to have more of a shrinking effect. When I examined him recently, his piles had completely healed leaving only a few little skin tags around the anus which are of no significance and should be left alone.

Piles can be both distressing and embarrassing. Many people will put up with them for years rather than go to the doctors, especially if they are worried about the prospect of an operation. With effective, simple therapies, however, all this suffering can be relieved without any threat of the surgeon's knife!

TREATMENT PLAN FOR PILES

Type

Internal
Prolapsed temporarily
Prolapsed permanently

↓

Investigations

Inspection
Palpitation
Protoscopy
Sigmoidoscopy

↓

Initial treatment

High-fibre diet
Anti-inflammatory suppositories
Bulking laxative

↓

Treatment of persistent symptoms

Conventional medicine	Homoeopathy	Herbalism
Anal stretching	Aloes	Pilewort cream
Haemorrhoidectomy	Hamamelis	Witch hazel
Injection	Hypericum	Yarrow
	Nux vomica	
	Pulsatilla	

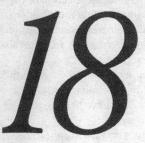

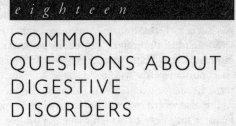

chapter
eighteen

COMMON QUESTIONS ABOUT DIGESTIVE DISORDERS

T he main problems which can upset the digestive system, as food passes through it, have been covered in this book. Inevitably, a few questions may still remain unanswered. While these may not relate to serious medical conditions, they are distressing for the affected person. A selection of the questions I am most frequently asked in the surgery are listed below.

My tongue has a continual coating on it and I have tried every mouthwash that is available. Is there something wrong with my stomach or could it be due to the type of food I eat?

A white or yellow coating on the tongue is not the sign of a disease. It consists of minute particles of food debris and bacteria. The coating is most noticeable first thing in the morning and is formed by smoking, breathing through the mouth and fasting. The latter two, dry up saliva in the mouth and are the reason why we develop a furred tongue when we have a high temperature. People with a cold or sinus problems nearly always have a coated tongue, as they inhale air through their mouths, drying their mouths. The coating is usually temporary. The furring will not rub off, but disappears naturally. Smoking must be stopped and every effort made to breathe through the nose rather than the mouth. Regular eating will stimulate the flow of saliva. An antiseptic mouthwash should also be used.

A black, hairy tongue is the result of a secondary fungal infection of the mouth usually after antibiotic therapy or, occasionally, when the patient is very run down. It is quite harmless and usually resolves spontaneously. However, it can be long standing and horrible to look at. An anti-fungal gel, such as Daktarin, will produce a rapid resolution.

Sometimes the tongue can develop a coating which is associated with mouth ulcers. These usually develop at times of emotional distress and heal spontaneously within ten days. Various creams have been tried but these have not been shown to speed the recovery.

It is also worth mentioning that normal tongues do vary in appearance. Fissures may develop which make the tongue look rather like a road map ('geographical tongue'). This is perfectly normal.

I am worried that my breath smells and am certain that people move away from me when I am talking. The trouble is I, myself, can't tell whether there is a smell or not. I try breathing into my hands and it seems alright but I read somewhere you can't smell your own breath.

It would be simple if we could smell the air we exhale instead of relying on a friend to tell us. If someone breathes over us the air goes straight up our nostrils stimulating the part of the nose responsible for the sense of smell. Unfortunately the odour only lasts for a few milliseconds, so if we breathe into our cupped hands in an attempt to smell our own breath, the odour will have dispersed by the time we sniff it. First, let's consider the causes:

- **Breathing through the mouth** Nearly everyone suffers from bad breath (halitosis) on waking in the morning. This is caused by sleeping with an open mouth, which dries the air we exhale giving it a fetid odour. A blocked nose or sinusitis will produce the same effect. Some people may just breathe through their mouth out of habit.
- **Food** Onions, garlic and alcohol are the main culprits although many other foods produce less intense odours. The lungs help to remove waste products from the body but this occurs some hours later after the digestion and absorption of food into the bloodstream. One patient of mine always chews raw garlic when she is ill. This is an excellent remedy but the smell can be offensive to other people. Another lady rubs garlic cloves into the soles of her feet and this is also detectable on her breath.

- **Unhealthy teeth and gums** Dental caries (caused by poor or irregular brushing), unhealthy gums (which are swollen and bleed easily) and rotting pockets of food between the teeth, can all produce halitosis.
- **Dyspepsia** A raised level of acid in the stomach from an unhealthy, high-fat diet produces sour-smelling breath.
- **Illness** Any condition affecting a large organ in the body can cause bad breath. Liver disease is the classic example. However, smelly breath on its own is not indicative of a serious illness.

If you are worried about halitosis, take these simple steps to ensure you avoid having it:

- It is easy to banish early morning halitosis by taking a drink or cleaning your teeth. Both will moisten the air as we breathe out. If you habitually breathe through your mouth, concentrate on keeping it closed all the time and try to breathe through your nose. Daily nasal salt washouts (a pinch of salt in a tumbler of water) will clear a blocked nose caused by a cold or sinusitis.
- As far as food is concerned, the only solution is to avoid those that are detectable on the breath.
- Dental hygiene is vital, especially in our so-called civilised society where food is refined and lacking in roughage. Chewing has a cleansing effect on the teeth which is lost when soft foods are bolted down. Too much sugar provides a rich medium for the growth of bacteria with their smelly toxins. To avoid this you need to eat plenty of roughage and omit sugar, biscuits and cakes. Even if an apple a day doesn't keep the doctor away, it will help to keep the dentist away as the citric acid helps to destroy bacteria in the mouth. This may be all that is needed to clear your halitosis.
- Inflammation of the gums (gingivitis) can arise from overzealous brushing and is often associated with a low intake of vitamin C. One 1000 mg tablet a day is needed to maintain healthy gums.
- To remove the sour smell due to a high stomach acid level, cut down on white sugar, white bread, refined flour, fried foods, animal fats and alcohol. Increase your intake of salads, fresh fruit, polyunsaturated fat and eat plenty of fibre. Aim for calmer, less rushed mealtimes and chew your food slowly.

In the vast majority of cases, the steps outlined above will restore the breath to its pleasant natural smell. However, if you are still not certain, a homoeopathic remedy can be added. Any one of the following remedies can be useful (taken in 6c):

- **Kreosotum** for gingivitis where the gums are inflamed, spongy and bleed easily;
- **Nux vomica** for sour-smelling breath due to dyspepsia;
- **Chelidonium** when the tongue has a thick yellow coating.

The breath-freshening mouthwash business is now a multi-million pound industry. The main ingredients are mint and the chemical actizol. As an alternative to these expensive, commercial preparations, I have found several herbal mixtures that give breath a pleasant odour:

- **Rosemary** An infusion of rosemary is prepared by pouring a cupful of boiling water over a teaspoon of the crushed herb. Cover and leave to infuse for ten minutes. Then use half as a mouthwash and drink the rest;
- **Thyme** Boil a sprig of thyme in a cupful of water for two to three seconds. Cover and steep for ten minutes. Again, use half the mixture as a mouthwash and drink the remainder;
- **Peppermint** Make a cup of peppermint tea with a tea bag, or infuse one teaspoon of fresh (or dried) leaves in a cupful of boiling water. Add a little freshly squeezed lemon juice. It is best to drink the tea as it counteracts the acidity in the stomach but you can also use it as a mouthwash to give the breath a pleasant minty smell.

By preventing the causes of halitosis and by using one of these herbal remedies you should be able to go out, confident that your breath smells clean and sweet. But if you must eat spicy or garlic laden food, then take pity on your friends and either chew fresh parsley leaves or keep your distance!

I always seem to have an itchy bottom. It drives me crazy when I'm out in company because I'm desperate to scratch myself. What can I do?

In medicine, the simplest reason for a given condition, is usually the one which is causing the problem. In ninety nine per cent of cases, an itchy bottom is caused by inefficient perineal cleaning. Faeces can lurk in the furrowed skin around the anus and, combined with moisture and sweat, it can serve to break down the normal resistance of the skin. The irritation leads to scratching, which abrades the surface. Once this surface layer is broken, it becomes a host to bacteria and fungi. At this point, the patient applies lotions, ointments and creams usually recommended by friends or chemists. Some of these damage the area further, producing an eczema-like rash. The irritation can be cleared by following a few basic principles:

- The area should be gently washed every morning, before retiring at night and after every bowel movement. Soap should be used sparingly, as the perfume can irritate the skin;
- Alternatively, moistened toilet tissues can be used (available from most supermarkets;
- Nylon underwear should be avoided, to reduce sweating. Wearing loose fitting trousers or skirts will help the skin to breathe;
- Try to identify the foods that cause anal irritation and avoid them;
- The bowels should be opened regularly without straining. Any constipation is best treated by increasing fibre intake or using a bulking laxative like Fybogel;
- The initial excoriated area can be quickly cleared using a conventional cream like Nystaform HC or Daktacort.

Haemorrhoids can also produce an itchy anal area as they increase mucus production and these should be dealt with (see Chapter 17). Very occasionally diabetes may cause pruritus, so a urine sample should be tested for evidence of excess sugar.

I've developed terrible wind which is most embarrassing when I'm out in company. Can I do anything about it?

Excessive flatulence is not only most unpleasant to the sufferer, but also antisocial. As well as producing belching and flatus, too much wind can cause colic, abdominal bloating and borborygmi (a constant rumbling of the stomach). Ninety nine per cent of the gas in the digestive system is composed of oxygen, nitrogen, hydrogen and methane. These are produced in different ways: swallowed air is the major source of oxygen and nitrogen, whereas bacteria in the intestines produce the hydrogen and methane. The nasty smell of flatus occurs when these four elements react together. As there are no bacteria in the stomach, very little gas is produced there. Patients who complain of belching almost invariably have been swallowing too much air. This is often a feature of anxiety. It also occurs in people who suffer from heartburn or indigestion, as they keep swallowing saliva in order to neutralise the stomach acid which has refluxed into the oesophagus and imitated it. Chewing gum, eating and drinking too quickly, and mouth ulcers can also encourage air ingestion. While most of this is belched, some may pass on into the intestines.

Strangely, people who complain of abdominal distension, pain and excess flatus have not been shown to have excess intestinal gas. The problem is in fact their inability to accommodate normal volumes of gas without pain. Where there is a very slow transit time through the gut, gas tends to collect at the corners of the large intestines. This is a common feature in irritable bowel syndrome (see Chapter 12).

The curing of excess wind therefore depends on treating the underlying anxiety and correcting any factors which encourage the swallowing of air. Although excessive production of gas is not primarily responsible for the condition, measures to reduce flatus formation should still be attempted.

- **Diet** Many jokes state that beans give rise to wind, but so do many other foodstuffs. Apples, raisins and bananas are common examples but perhaps the most lethal are grapes. Obviously, these are to be avoided, as should changing to a high-fibre diet too quickly. Eating plain live yoghurt or acidophilus tablets can also help.
- **Herbal treatment** Relief may be obtained by taking peppermint tea after meals. Hot parsley tea in 45 mls (three tablespoons) doses and chewing a sprig or two of parsley (or angelica) after a meal can be most effective. Mustard seeds can also be chewed in unlimited amounts. A tea made up of equal amounts of lemon balm and chamomile flowers, taken before each meal will improve flatulence of nervous origin. A number of cooking herbs, including rosemary, sage, and marjoram, contain essential oils that aid digestion. If used generously in cooking, they can help flatulence.

I seem to have constant problems with my stomach. Sometimes it is wind, at others I just feel bloated. Basically, it is a general feeling that my stomach is unsettled. My bowels are erratic, varying between constipation and diarrhoea. I can't eat big meals and have constant indigestion. What should I do?

I think we all know the feeling when our stomachs feel unsettled or not quite right. Usually this sensation passes after a few days but some people suffer almost continously and this can be most distressing. I am convinced the problem is that our meals contain too great a variety of foods, making it more difficult for the digestive system to cope with them. The solution is to eat more simply, avoiding rich foods.

We often need to look back to the past for the answer to our digestive problems because it is only in the latter part of this century that food has become so refined, with so many additives. In 1891 an American doctor called William Hay became ill with stomach problems and his American colleagues were unable to help him. He decided to cure himself by drastically modifying his diet. He coined the phrase 'fundamental eating' which was based on consuming only natural foods in modest quantities and not mixing different foodstuffs. After making a complete recovery from his supposedly untreatable illness, Hay changed his entire way of practising medicine and devoted his time to treating patients by dietary change. The Hay diet, as it is now called, is perfectly safe and applicable to anyone, of any age. There are five basic rules you need to follow:

- Starches and sugars should not be mixed together with protein and acid fruits in the same meal;
- Vegetables, fruits and salads should form a major part of your food intake;
- Fats should be eaten only in small quantities;
- Only wholegrain and unprocessed starches should be used, omitting all refined and processed foods. In particular, white flour, sugar and all foods which are made with them should be avoided, as well as highly processed fats (such as margarine);
- There should be an interval of at least four hours between meals.

This diet will certainly help all those of you with severe digestive problems. The millions of sufferers with low-grade, non-specific symptoms, will also be surprised at the immediate benefits this approach will bring. Many of my patients have adopted the Hay diet and have seen dramatic results.

I know that additives in food can upset the digestive system but which ones should I look out for? It would take hours to go round a supermarket looking at every tin and bottle!

So much is written on the subject of food additives and it is not known how harmful they really are. On one hand, naturopaths advise you not to eat foodstuffs with any additives in them and on the other, the food industry claims they do no harm at all. The answer probably lies somewhere in the middle. I agree with the person who asked this question – it is absolutely impossible to check everything you buy. My advice is to try and avoid the additives that have definitely been shown, in some people, to cause a reaction. In my own practice, patients who have been to the allergy clinic at the local hospital have tested positive to the following:

- **E 102** Tartrazine (an orange food colourant);
- **E 210, 211** Benzoic acids;
- **E 220, 221, 223, 224** Sulphite based preservatives;
- **E 250, 251** Nitrite preservatives;
- **E 310, 320, 321** Anti-oxidants;
- **E 621, 622, 623** Monosodium glutamate and related flavour enhancers.

At first glance, even this seems a long list. Rather than examining everything on the supermarket shelves, it is better to note which upsets your stomach, at home. Look at what you have just eaten, check which additives it contained and avoid these in the future. It is amazing how little time it takes to learn which foods contain the particular additives.

Is there really any connection between children's behaviour and what they eat?

It can be difficult to draw the line between the behaviour of a child that is within the normal limits of high energy and one which is hyperactive. However, there is no doubt that, when certain additives are omitted from children's diets, their behaviour can dramatically improve. You should also bear in mind that hyperactivity can be the result of a brain disorder or a psychological disturbance.

It is now accepted that E 102 (tartrazine) is toxic to children. This is present in many squashes and sweets. You may find changing to fruit juice beneficial. E 621 (monosodium glutamate) has also been shown to cause sickness and abdominal bloating. America is well ahead of the rest of us with regards to avoiding food additives. Their supermarkets now have whole shelves devoted to monosodium glutamate-free foods.

As a general rule, if your child's behaviour is suspect, then it is well worth eliminating as many additives as possible (see list on page 202) although this may seem a near-impossible task! If their behaviour does not improve, it is important to seek qualified medical advice.

I have suffered with lower abdominal pain for several months and whenever I go to my doctors he simply says I have intermittent colic and there is nothing I can do about it. I've only ever heard colic mentioned in relation to babies. Is mine a different type? Is there anything I can do about it?

Colic is an acutely painful spasm in any part of the digestive system, although it is most common in the large intestine. The pain is not constant but comes and goes in waves. Several conditions can produce this spasm including excess wind, irritable bowel syndrome (see pages 125–150), colitis, diverticulitis (see pages 151–160) and gastro-enteritis. In these situations, the muscle in the bowel becomes irritated and twitchy, causing pain. Constipation (see pages 91–106), intestinal obstruction or a gall stone blocking the bile duct (see pages 80–90), all produce severe colic as the body tries to overcome the obstruction.

Colic in babies is frequently associated with wind but it has been shown that bottle-fed babies are more likely to suffer. Breast-fed babies, whose mothers consume large quantities of cow's milk have a far higher incidence of colic than babies whose mothers drink little or no milk. A connection with food allergy should not, therefore, be overlooked. Whatever the cause, the muscle of the intestine wall becomes very sensitive and contracts unnecessarily, producing acute discomfort which makes the baby cry.

- **Conventional treatment** is with painkillers and antispasmodics. Wherever possible, the underlying condition should be tackled. In babies, paracetamol syrup (for example Calpol) is effective coupled with a change to soya milk in case there is an allergy to cow's milk. Antispasmodics cannot be used in infants, because of the risk of suppressing the baby's breathing.
- **Herbal treatment** in adults includes the following teas, all of which ease colic: chamomile, peppermint, catmint or seed teas. All are commercially available, and the choice depends on personal preference. My own, however, is for an infusion of fennel, aniseed and caraway seeds. These should be mixed

together in equal parts: 5 mls (one teaspoon) of the mixed ingredients are crushed and added to a cupful of boiling water. This is covered for ten minutes, strained and drunk hot. Tincture of ginger in hot, sweetened water will relieve pain and disperse flatulence. An infusion of powdered ginger taken warm in 15 mls (one tablespoon) doses will also relieve colic. Peppermint oil and liquorice are known for their antispasmodic properties. Infant colic can be relieved by any of these herbal remedies given warm in 5 mls (one teaspoon) doses.

- **Homoeopathic remedies** are particularly effective for colic and are invaluable in babies, as there is no risk of side-effects. Chamomilla is my treatment of choice for infants, either as a small tablet, dissolved under the tongue or as granules, which can be chewed. Colocynth is used for pain which is brought on by anger and feels better for pressure on the abdomen. It is also good for cutting pains. The patient may also feel very restless. Ipecacuanha is best for colic associated with nausea and vomiting. Magnesia phosphorica is excellent for sharp pains that are better for heat. Nux vomica is for colic associated with overindulgence in alcohol and fatty spicy food. Constipation is also common in such cases.

Colic can be a real nuisance but will settle down with careful treatment. I shall never forget the sleepless nights spent with my first baby until we discovered Chamomilla. It was such a relief!

I seem very prone to an upset stomach, especially at times of stress. It usually clears up in two or three days but always leaves me with a loss of appetite which can take weeks to recover. Is there anything I can do to stop this?

Most appetite loss, except for anorexia nervosa, is a result either of physical illness, for example mouth ulcers, tooth problems, many digestive disorders and acute infections. It is a common result of high fever and any condition which causes nausea and vomiting. It can also be a side-effect of drug therapy. Times of stress may cause a marked decrease in appetite. While in some people, worry and tension make them eat more, in others the desire for food is lost.

Once the underlying condition has cleared, the appetite usually returns to normal. In some cases, as for the person who asked this question, a delay occurs leading to a vicious circle of increasingly poor nutrition. Any food that is taken in must therefore be of high nutritional value (high in calories, vitamins and minerals, low in bulk). Avoid fatty food, so go mainly for freshly-made fruit and vegetable juices, puréed soups made from briefly cooked ingredients and plenty of yoghurt. Small, frequent meals are better than three meals a day. As an insurance against deficiency, vitamin B complex should be taken before meals together with 15 mg of zinc chelate.

While conventional medicine has nothing to offer to stimulate the appetite, both herbal and homoeopathic treatments are effective. During acute illness, appetite loss is the body's natural response, so attempts to stimulate it will not be effective and are contra indicated. When the initial symptoms have subsided, a decoction of gentian root, poplar bark, meadowsweet herb and century herb (in equal parts) can be taken in doses of 45 ml (three tablespoons) three times daily. Although this sounds complicated, once you have bought the four herbs, it is almost as simple as making a cup of tea. Alternatively, an infusion of sweet cecily herb in the same dose will both restore appetite and act as a tonic. For emotional problems, a cupful of peppermint tea, in place of normal tea, can be most helpful.

Usually one of the following homoeopathic remedies work quickly but if they are not successful, then it will be necessary to choose a remedy which is compatible with the individual's personality (consult a qualified practitioner). These remedies include:

- **Lycopodium** when hunger is present initially but the appetite is lost after a mouthful or two;
- **Pulsatilla** for lack of thirst and an aversion to fatty, rich food;
- **Lignatia** for complete loss of appetite from grief, worry or tension;
- **Rhus tox** for total loss of appetite following a digestive upset.

Every time I go out for a meal, I develop an attack of hiccups. This can be most embarrassing especially if I am in company.

While not serious, hiccups are a common problem. Hiccups occur as a result of a spasm in the diaphragm, caused by the irritation in the nerves that supply it. As the diaphragm contracts, air is involuntarily and rapidly breathed in and the vocal cords snap shut. This produces the characteristic, uncontrollable, loud noise. Hiccups are usually triggered by gas in the stomach, which makes the stomach distend and exerts pressure on the nerves of the diaphragm. The most common reason for the extra gas is eating a bigger meal than usual (when we go to a restaurant or a friend's house for dinner, for example). Hiccups are also common in children, usually from the excessive consumption of fizzy drinks.

Most attacks of hiccups are short-lived and can be prevented by eating smaller meals. However, in persistent cases, the most effective way to get rid of them is to lie on your back on the floor and bring your knees up to your chest, holding them there for a count of three and then relaxing. This puts pressure on the diaphragm and stops the spasms. Obviously this can only be carried out at home. Even drinking out of the opposite side of a glass may be difficult in company. In these circumstances simply holding your breath (which prevents the sudden inhalation of air) can break up the run of hiccups.

In a number of people hiccups can last for several hours or very occasionally, even longer. Orthodox medicine has little to offer in such cases – mainly sedatives to suppress the hiccup reflex.

A herbalist colleague of mine recommends chewing fresh mint leaves or dill seeds. Gripe water, which is used to treat colic in babies, contains dill and may therefore be effective. Alternatively, place one teaspoon of crushed dill seeds in a little hot water. Stir, infuse for a few minutes and then strain. Cold water is then added and the mixture drunk.

I am thirty four years old and have been overweight as long as I can remember. Up until last year, I didn't worry about it, as my husband was also a bit on the fat side. Recently he has started going to the local gym as he says being too heavy is bad for you and causes all sorts of illnesses. He has now lost nearly two stone and keeps telling me to go on a diet. The trouble is, everything I eat seems to make me put on weight. Is there something wrong with my digestion? What would you advise me to do?

We live in an affluent society where we eat far too much. The limit on our eating seems only to depend on the amount of money in our pockets. Heart attacks and strokes have been linked to obesity. It also predisposes the sufferer to a range of other problems: arthritis, back pain, haemorrhoids, varicose veins, high blood pressure and cholesterol levels. Obesity can prevent people from taking part in sporting activities and reduce their overall efficiency. So my advice to this lady is, for her own sake, to lose weight. The formula is simple: if you eat more calories than you need, then you put on weight. The only problem with this is that we are all different. In some people, digestive systems are super efficient, absorbing absolutely everything from our food. In others, the breakdown and absorption of food is not as effective and many of the calories pass through into the bowel. This helps to explain why two members of the same family, on the same diet, can be totally different in body shape (one may be slim and the other fat).

Many people claim they are overweight because of their 'glands'. This is a total myth. The thyroid gland is underactive, leading to weight gain, in very rare cases – I only see four or five a year. Some drugs (particularly steroids, oral contraceptives and hormone replacements) may also cause obesity. Having said this, the vast majority of obese people are overweight because they eat too much, although they may be reluctant to admit it. I do not wish to sound unsympathetic, as losing weight can be very difficult. For this reason, I usually offer a course of acupuncture or self-hypnosis to accompany a low calorie diet. Acupuncture will reduce the intense desire to eat, especially when used in combination with a regime of exercise and sound nutrition. Small, metal studs are placed in the ears. They are then taped and can be stimulated by the wearer, whenever a compulsion to eat afflicts them.

Hypnosis is used initially to build up an aversion to food. Self-hypnosis can then be practised every time there is a desire to eat. Some people may become overweight through overeating out of unhappiness. In such cases, self-hypnosis can improve low self-esteem and poor self-image.

I am nearly halfway through my first pregnancy and am gaining too much weight. I am worried that if I go on a diet the baby will suffer. What nutrients does the baby need and how can I lose weight without harming it?

Weight gain must be watched carefully throughout pregnancy and should not be allowed to creep beyond normal limits. As a rough guide you should aim to put on no more than 21 lb over the nine months. This consists of 7 lb for the baby; 7 lb for the uterus, placenta and fluid surrounding the baby and 7 lb for the increased volume of blood and breast size.

When you are pregnant, however, two major changes happen to the digestive system. First, there is an increase in the amount of enzymes that break food down and second, the passage of food through the gut slows down. Both of these changes are designed to increase the amount of food absorbed into the bloodstream, ensuring the growing baby receives sufficient nourishment. This system works well until we eat too much and the excess is turned into fat. It is necessary, therefore, to choose food which is rich in nutrients, benefiting both the mother and baby, without leading to excessive weight gain.

The nutrients needed to do this include:

- **Calcium**, which is found in cereals, pulses, green vegetables, nuts and sardines. Although cow's milk is a good source of calcium, research has shown that, if a pregnant woman drinks milk or eats dairy products made with cow's milk, the baby is more likely to develop dermatitis and eczema;
- **Iron** found in offal, black pudding, green vegetables, cereals and dried apricots;
- **Vitamin A** from oily fish, fish liver oil, orange vegetables and fruit (carrots, yellow melons, peaches and tomatoes, for example);
- **Vitamin C** found in leafy green vegetables, most other vegetables and fruit (especially green peppers, strawberries, blackcurrants, guavas and citrus fruit);
- **Vitamin D** found in oily fish and fish liver oil. If you are lucky enough to be pregnant in summer, then sunshine will produce this vitamin naturally;
- **Folic acid** which is in leafy green vegetables, liver and wheatgerm.

If you ensure you eat plenty of these types of food, along with a limited amount of carbohydrate and protein, then the baby will receive everything it needs and the mother will not gain excess weight. Gentle exercise every day will help you control your weight.

I am ten weeks pregnant and have been sick constantly for the past five weeks. Every time I eat or drink something my stomach throws it straight back. Is there anything that will help?

Over fifty per cent of pregnant women experience vomiting in the first three months of pregnancy. Although this commonly occurs in the morning, it can just as well happen at any other time of the day or night. The exact reason for pregnancy sickness is not really known although it is assumed to be the effect of the sudden hormone changes on the stomach lining. Normally, if the mother is well-nourished, morning sickness will not deprive the baby of any nutrients.

If you are suffering from morning sickness, try eating frequent, small meals. A cup of tea with some dry toast or unsweetened wholemeal biscuits on waking, often helps to clear the initial nausea. Avoiding fatty, greasy foods, coffee, strong tea and alcohol, while ensuring a well-balanced diet (with protein, for example nuts, seeds, grains and pulses) will also be beneficial.

The risk to the unborn baby in taking orthodox drugs for this condition, far outweighs any benefit to the expectant mother. However, some of the herbal and homoeopathic treatments are most effective:

- **Chamomile tea** is the first herbal remedy to try. Drink a warm cupful at bedtime made from three to four tablespoons of the herb, steamed with a pint of water. The same mixture should be sipped in the morning. Some women find raspberry leaf tea helpful, whereas others prefer peppermint;
- **Nux vomica** for sickness associated with irritability, constipation and a brown tongue. I find this is the preparation I prescribe in most cases;
- **Pulsatilla** for weepiness and a white tongue;
- **Tabacum** for constant nausea and sickness all day;
- **Sepia** for nausea on smelling food, associated with chilliness, irritability and prolonged, low abdominal pain;
- **Argentum nit** where there is craving for sweets and excessive flatulence. It best suits the apprehensive person who has a tendency to panic;
- **Ipecacuanha** for continual nausea, vomiting of bile, diarrhoea, lack of thirst and irritability.

Morning sickness may also be relieved by vitamin B6 (up to 100 mg daily) for a short period, preferably in conjunction with magnesium (300 mg daily).

My son is nine years old and I have had to pick him up from school several times because he has been crying with stomach pains. I have taken him to see my doctor and he has told me it must be a problem at school. His teacher, however, says he is a happy boy with plenty of friends and thinks there must be a problem at home. The pain is mainly down his left side and doesn't make him sick. I'm not sure what to do next.
The difficulty, in this situation, is deciding whether the pain is from an actual physical illness or whether it is psychological. It is undoubtedly a common problem. Surveys show that over ten per cent of children, between three and fourteen years of age, suffer with an attack of abdominal pain every month. In my experience, there is little doubt that many of these children have an emotional problem. However, it is dangerous for a doctor to form this opinion without careful consideration of the type and nature of the pain.

Let us consider the features of physical and psychological abdominal pain:

- **The site of the pain** Psychological pain is nearly always located around the navel area or just above it. Pain in other regions is more likely to be physical. Urine infections present low, central abdominal tenderness. Pain in the loins is suggestive of a kidney infection. If the pain is on either side and low down then it may arise from the intestines or from the ovaries (in a girl);
- **Duration** Pain which is continuous and keeps the child awake at night or, more significantly, wakes a child up during sleep, should be regarded as physical. Psychological pain often only lasts between fifteen minutes and one hour, and rarely affects sleep;
- **Type of pain** Children often find it difficult to describe the type of pain they are experiencing. It is particularly important to discover if the pain is colicky in nature (where the discomfort comes and goes in waves, building up to a peak and then subsiding). If this is the case, there is likely to be a physical cause;
- **Precipitating factors** It is important for your doctor to identify any obvious cause by direct questioning. Most children will not admit to any underlying anxiety or stress and teachers are reluctant to concede there are any problems in the child/teacher relationship. A child's anxieties and stresses at school, can often be missed because parents and teachers feel that, if the child is making good progress and is a high achiever, then there is no problem. Academic success, however, is not a good guideline and if the child is specifically asked about school work, bullying, arguments at home, teasing at school and fears regarding other pupils and staff, they will often volunteer information which may have a significant bearing on their illness;
- **Examination findings** A thorough examination, in the presence of the parents is essential. This has two purposes: to identify any underlying disease and, if none is present, to reassure both parents and child of the absence of any serious cause;
- **Investigations** Many parents want a simple test to prove a cause for the pain. However, the only investigation of help (as all other tests are invariably negative in cases such as these) is a urine sample to rule out an infection.

After considering all the above features, I am usually certain whether the pain is physical or psychological. However, the child in the original question, complained of pain down the left hand side of the abdomen, which immediately made me suspicious of an underlying physical cause. On closer questioning, he admitted to some diarrhoea, which tended to come on before the pain started, and forced him to ask to go to the toilet during class. It had also made his teacher think that it was all due to some emotional upset as many people associate diarrhoea with 'nerves'. While this can be true, his mother maintained that she thought it unlikely it was psychological and this, coupled with the site of the pain, further heightened my suspicions.

The child was not ill, so I was confident there was no serious cause to his pain and in my own mind the diagnosis lay in irritable bowel syndrome or food allergy. A recent study showed that one in eight cases of irritable bowel syndrome in adults, had suffered with recurrent abdominal pain in childhood, some four times more than those without IBS. This diagnosis should be considered in any child with abdominal pain with associated bowel disturbance and particularly, as in this case, if the onset of pain is heralded by increased or looser bowel movements. A similar number of children have pain associated with food intolerance or allergy. The pain is usually left-sided and may also occur with diarrhoea. However, there are nearly always other signs, including a variety of skin disorders or asthma.

If irritable bowel syndrome is the cause of a child's pain, then unfortunately there is no definite test to prove it. It may also have a psychological cause but, in my experience, this is uncommon. I explained carefully there was nothing seriously wrong with his stomach, as children of that age do need strong reassurance. I suggested to his mum to increase the fibre in his diet gradually. This normally removes the pain and diarrhoea of IBS in children. I am pleased to say that since then he has not had any further discomfort.

USEFUL ADDRESSES

> **IMPORTANT**
> There are many excellent alternative therapists across the UK. It is worth writing to the official associations for the names in your area.

The Council for Acupuncture
179 Gloucester Place
London NW1 6DX

British Hypnosis Research
The School of Health and Community Studies
University of Derby
Western Road
Mickleover
Derby DE3 5GX

The Society of Homoeopaths
2 Artizan Road
Northampton
NN1 4HU

General Council and Register of Consultant Herbalists
18 Sussex Square
Brighton
East Sussex
BN2 5AA

The Coeliac Society
PO Box 220
High Wycombe
Buckinghamshire
HP11 2HY

The IBS Network
(General Enquiries)
St John's House
Hither Green Hospital
London SE13 6RU
Tel: 0181 698 4611

(Gut Reaction Newsletter and Membership)
Northern General Hospital
Sheffield
S5 7AU
Tel: 0114 261 1531

INDEX

abdominal distension, 147–8
abdominal pain, 28, 171–5, 210–12
aconite, 117
acupressure, 14, 102, 122, 158
acupuncture, 12–15, 48–9, 65, 86–8, 102,
    119–21, 145, 158, 168, 208
addresses, 213–14
adrenalin, 136–7
aesculus, 146, 193
agrimony, 119, 164
alcohol, 36, 54, 111
allergies, 68–9
aloes, 48, 117, 194
alternative therapies, 12–19 *and passim*
alumina, 100
American cranesbill, 48
anaemia, 76
angelica, 148, 201
aniseed, 204
anorexia nervosa, 56–7
antacids, 28, 43
antibiotics, 44, 53, 115, 190
Anusol, 190
appendicitis, 10, 55
Argentum nit, 47, 117, 210
arrowroot, 147
Arsenicum album, 31, 64, 117, 164, 168
aspirin, 53, 54

bad breath, 197–9
barium tests, 25, 39–40, 59, 95, 154–5
basil, 146, 148
bay, 48
behaviour of children, 203–5
belladonna, 145, 157
berberis, 89
bleeding, 188
blood tests, 59, 77, 113
bryonia, 157
bulimia nervosa, 57
bulking agents, 97–8

caffeine, 41
calcium, 209
calorie-controlled dieting, 4, 86
Calpol, 204

cancer, 176–85
    alternative therapy, 180–4
    management, 179–84
caraway, 48, 205
Carbenoxolone, 29, 30
carrot, 146
catmint, 48, 204
cecily, 206
celandine, 193
century, 48, 206
chamomile, 48, 64, 158, 201, 204, 205,
    210
charcoal, 146
Chelidonium, 199
chemotherapy, 180
chickweed, 164
China, 118
cider vinegar, 147
Cimetedine, 29, 30, 43
cinnamon, 148
cloves, 65
codeine, 115, 147
coeliac disease, 75–9
colic, 204–5
Colocynth, 118, 145, 157, 205
Colofac, 132
colonoscopy, 95
constipation, 55, 91–106, 129, 145–6
    alternative therapy, 99–102
    management, 96–106
co-proxamol, 53
coping, 140–2, 144–5
coriander, 48
counselling, 62, 131–2
Crohn's disease, 165–70

Daktarin, 197
dandelion, 48
diagnosis, 111–12, 123, 129–31, 171–2
diarrhoea, 10, 107–22, 129, 147
    alternative therapy, 116–22
    management, 114–22
diet, 3, 35, 62, 71, 77–9, 86, 96–7,
    133–5, 155–6, 165, 178, 181, 192,
    201
dieting, *see* calorie-controlled dieting

digestive problems
  in children, 104–5, 115–16
  incidence of, 2–3, 126
  reasons for, 3–4, 20–4, 35–8, 52–7, 91–3,
    108–11, 125, 177
digestive process, 6–11
dill, 207
Dioralyte, 115–16
diverticulitis, 125, 151–60
  alternative therapy, 155–60
  management, 155–60
Domperidone, 61
drugs, 28–30, 43–4, 61–2, 98–9, 114–16, 132–
  3, 137–8, 144, 155, 190–1, 204
Dulcamara, 118

ear problems, 56
endoscopy, 25, 40, 59
enemas, 95
exercise, 86, 96, 135–6, 164–5, 178, 181,
  192
explanation, 131–2

faecal impaction, 102–4
fennel, 48, 144, 204
figs, 146
flatulence, see wind
fluid intake, 97, see also hydration
folic acid, 209
food additives, 68–9, 202–3
food poisoning, 53
fringe tree, 89–90
Fybogel, 147, 190

gall stones, 54–5, 80–90
  alternative therapy, 86–90
  management, 84–90
garlic, 119
gastritis, 52–3
Gastrocote, 30
Gaviscon, 30
gentian, 206
geranium, 119
ginger, 64–5, 148, 205
graphites, 47
guelder rose, 102
gullet, see oesophagus

haemorrhoids, see piles
halitosis, 197–9
hamamelis, 193
Hay, William, 202
healthy eating, 5

heartburn, 20–34
herbal medicine, 19, 31–2, 48, 64–5, 89–90,
  101–2, 119, 144–5, 157–8, 164, 192,
  201, 204–5
  alternative therapy, 30–2
  management, 26–32
hiatus hernia, 23
hiccups, 206–7
history of patients, 130
homoeopathy, 16–17, 30–1, 47, 63–4, 88–9,
  100–1, 117–19, 145, 147, 156–7, 164,
  181, 193–4, 205
hops, 144
hydration, 114
hypericum, 194
hypnosis, 17–18, 45–6, 142, 158–60, 208

immune system, 68, 78, 116, 137, 164–5, 167,
  176–7, 180
Imodium, 147
inadequate digestion, 73–4
inflammatory bowel disease, 161–70
  management, 162–5, 167–70
infusions, 32
intestine, large, 10–11
intestine, small, 9–10, 74–9
intolerance of food, 69–70, 75, 133–5, 138
  management, 70–2
Ipecachuana, 205, 210
iron, 209
irritable bowel syndrome, 123–50, 212
  management, 131–60
ispaghula, 132

kaolin, 114
kreosotum, 199

lavender, 144
laxatives, 98–9, 146
lemon, 48, 144, 199, 201
Lignatia, 206
linseed, 102–2
liquorice, 146, 205
Loperamide, 115
Lycopodium, 31, 146, 206

magnesia phosphorica, 145, 157, 205
malabsorption, 73–9
  management, 77–9
marjoram, 48, 148, 201
marshmallow, 48
Maxolon, 29
meadowsweet, 31, 206

menstruation, 56
mercurius corr., 164, 168
Metoclopramide, 61
migraine, 56
mint, 145, 207, *see also* peppermint
morning sickness, 210
morphine, 114
Motilium, 132
mouth, 8
mustard, 148, 201

natrum sol, 147
naturopathy, 116–17, 144, 155–6
nausea, 52–66
nutmeg, 148
nux vomica, 31, 63, 100, 145, 193, 199, 205, 210

obesity, 3–4, 27–8
obstruction, 55
oesophagus, 9
Omeprazole, 29, 30

paracetamol, 204
parsley, 201
Pecac, 64
peppermint, 90, 148, 157, 199, 201, 204, 205, 206, 210
peritonitis, 40, 153
personality, change, 142–3
phenol, 190–1
phosphoric acid, 118
phosphorus, 31, 164, 168
piles, 185–95
    alternative therapy, 192–5
    management, 190–5
pilewort, 193
plumbum, 100
Podophyllum, 117–18, 147
poplar, 206
positive thinking, 182–3
pregnancy, 56, 208–9
Prenisolone, 163
prevention, 178
proctalgia fugax, 104
Proctosedyl, 190
prunes, 146
Pulsatilla, 47, 63, 118, 194, 206, 210

questions on digestive disorders, 196–212

radiotherapy, 180
raspberry, 210
reactions to food, 67–72
reflux, 20–2
Rehydrat, 115–16
rhubarb, 101
rhus tox, 206
rosemary, 48, 199, 201

sage, 201
self help, 62, 133–6, 138–9, 192–3
Sepia, 47, 210
Shigella, *see* diarrhoea
sigmoidoscopy, 113–14
slippery elm, 48, 158, 164
smoking, 36, 41, 178
sodium, 115
stomach, 9
stool sample, 112–13
stress, 36, 41–2, 45, 58, 60, 127, 136–43, 158, 164
    anti-stress plan, 139–41
Sulphasalazine, 163
sulphur, 100, 118, 147
surgery, 32, 73, 84–5, 111, 155, 180
symptoms, 38–9, 82–4, 126–9, 151–4, 176–7, 187–8

tabacum, 210
tests, 24–6, 39–40, 59–60, 77, 84, 93–5, 112–14, 130–1, 154–5, 162, 167, 179, 188–90
thyme, 48, 145, 199
thyroid problems, 56

ulcerative colitis, 161–5
ulcers, 35–51, 53, 161, 165
    alternative therapy, 45–9
    management, 40–9
ultrasound scanning, 59–60, 84

veratrum, 118
vitamins, 117, 165, 192, 209
vomiting, 52–66
    alternative therapy, 62–6
    management, 61–6

wind, 129, 147–8, 200–2
witch hazel, 193

yarrow, 193